A NEW CALM

A Story of Breakthrough Neuroscience Technology
Patented to Quickly and Naturally
Reduce Stress and Improve Performance

Michael Galitzer, M.D.
Larry Trivieri Jr.

Authors of
Outstanding Health

gatekeeper press

Disclaimer

The information in this book is not to be used to treat or diagnose any particular disease or any particular patient. Neither the authors nor the publisher is engaged in rendering professional advice or services to the individual reader. The ideas and recommendations in this book are not intended either as a substitute for professional health care advice or as a consultation with a professional health care provider. The publisher and authors are neither responsible nor liable for any adverse effects, losses, damages or other consequences arising from any information or recommendations in this book. All matters pertaining to your personal health should be supervised by a health care professional. Contact information given in this book was accurate at the time of printing.

Copyright © 2016 by Michael Galitzer and Larry Trivieri Jr.

All rights reserved. Published 2016.

Printed in the United States of America

Gatekeeper Press, Publisher
3971 Hover Road, Suite 77
Columbus, Ohio 43123--2839

ISBN 978-0-9971175-0-9

ISBN (e-book version) 978-0-9971175-1-6

NuCalm® is a registered trademark of Solace Lifesciences Inc.

Library of Congress Control Number: 2016962468

Cover design and photograph by Jon Pietz, Brand X

Edited by S. R. Dozier

The authors would like to thank the senior executive team of Solace Lifesciences for their selfless work in bringing NuCalm and this book to the world, including those not specified in the text: Chris Gross, chief operating officer, and Ashley Blanke, executive vice president of business development.

To Dr. G. Blake Holloway

for his tireless commitment to helping others heal

and for his many years of exploring and experimenting

to develop the NuCalm technology.

TABLE OF CONTENTS

FOREWORD

Life is energy. Everything about life is energy.

Energy fuels our state of being, both physical and emotional.

When emotions enter our life, our body's wiring changes.

That's my understanding of how we function.

If we want to have a vital life, we need to attain and sustain pure, positive energy. That is the most important thing we can do for our body. This is not a *should*, it is the *must*.

The quality of your life depends on the energy you put in and the energy you take out. Regardless of where you're at in life, or what your goals for the future are, if you are exhausted and stressed, you won't have the energy and passion you need to achieve results.

We all know that how you feel is influenced by your thoughts, and that you can control those thoughts. What's fascinating is how your mind works with your brain to govern your body's physical, mental and emotional state, from health and happiness to disease and fear.

Think about how your brain works. The human brain is two million years old. Your brain is not designed to make you happy—that is your job. Your brain is wired for survival. It gets signals from your autonomic nervous system, and sends out commands to the body through the two autonomic branches: the sympathetic and the para-sympathetic nervous systems.

Your brain is always looking around for what's wrong, and if there's a threat, the sympathetic "fight or flight" response immediately kicks in. That's our basic survival response that's kept the human race going since cave man times. In today's world, this response serves us well when we're crossing a busy intersection, but it does not serve us if we permanently live in that emotional state, always fearing what danger might lurk around the corner.

Since there are no saber-toothed tigers for us to deal with anymore, we pollute our mind with negative stories. We worry about what people are thinking about us, or if we make enough money, or our relationships. The problem is that we get stuck in that response, and that can hurt both our body and our outlook.

It's a classic case of "as you think, so you become."

The secret is learning how to let go of these stories that you're stressing yourself about, so you can handle the real problems from a place of total energy. When you're feeling tired or stressed or upset, it's difficult to make good decisions.

I'm known as someone who makes big demands on my mind and body, and someone who is always in constant sympathetic overload. I've driven myself to constantly look forward, seeking better ways to find the energy I need to create a vital life.

My goal is to help you have more energy than you've ever had, and sustain it with as little effort as possible. Over the years, I have been obsessed with sharing the many tools and methods I've discovered to help you build an energy base, challenge it, expand it and create a momentum that fuels you to be your best self.

Over the course of time, though, experience has taught me that I can continue to ask a lot from my body *and* I can continue to drive to achieve my goals—but that is only possible if I have *balance*.

What I have learned is that if I can balance the parasympathetic and the sympathetic nervous systems, I can sustain longer, I can keep a high level of health and I can maintain a high level of achievement. I need that balance. Without it, I can't sustain the pace.

We all need balance. We can't just drive, drive, drive, drive and drive. We have to understand this concept. There has to be balance in the autonomic nervous system. With that balance, there is vitality, relaxation and enjoyment. Once you experience this sort of vibrant health and energy in your life, you will never want to go back.

As I was learning this lesson about achieving balance in my life, I was privileged to have Dr. Michael Galitzer as my physician. He told me about a new technology that might help me, called NuCalm. I tried it for the first time at his office in Los Angeles in early May 2015. I loved how restored, how rejuvenated and how focused I felt afterward.

NuCalm is the most powerful technology I have ever used, or

heard of, to balance the autonomic nervous system. When I say used or heard of, I'm not saying I simply convinced myself that this is a great technology. I read the research and the evaluations by some the world's leading experts, so I *know* it's a great technology.

I live in six different locations, am on stage for 12-plus hours at a time at events, and often get as little as four hours of sleep a night. Needless to say, my schedule can be grueling—but I'm pulled to it, not pushed to it. I use NuCalm as a tool to make up for the sleep debt my lifestyle creates. It restores my balance and allows me to produce results. If I have just 20 minutes before I have to go on stage, instead of exercising, power napping or eating, I'll get on NuCalm. It completely focuses me, energizes me and allows me to be at my best on stage.

When you are in balance like this, everything is in sync. You're in that flow state. The perfect words come to you, and you're like "Where did that come from?" When stress disappears, you come up with that brilliant idea you've been trying to find. You're in the zone, and with NuCalm, you can put yourself in the zone instead of hoping the zone shows up.

Most people have created their own highway to stress, upset and worry, while they have a dirt road to happiness. It's neurological. The more you go into a certain state, the more you go into it automatically. You've met people who are always upset or worried. You've met those people who tell terrible jokes, but they enjoy them so much that they crack you up, too. So, we prime, or wire, ourselves to be a certain way. The more you use NuCalm, the easier it will be for you to prime yourself for balance and to deal more effectively with the challenges that arise in your life.

If you want to achieve maximum success, whether it's in business, at home, with your children or your spouse, with your friends, or with your health, you have to be able to manage stress. You must have balance and you must have commitment, strength and positive energy.

Basically, you can live your life in one of two ways. You can let your mind and brain run you the way they have in the past. You can let them flash any picture or sound or feeling, and you can respond automatically on cue, like Pavlov's dog responding to a bell. Or, you can consciously choose balance, restoration and performance.

NuCalm is the tool for creating balance in your mind and body. I highly recommend that you check it out as a predictable, safe and effective technology to manage your stress, improve your sleep quality and provide a foundation for massive success. By doing it every day, you literally train your nervous system to function at its best.

When I see a company with a product that has so much promise and can do so much good for humanity, it's easy for me to get behind it. I've been telling anybody who will listen about NuCalm since I started using it. They all love it.

Let's face it. No one is getting any younger, right? Every one of us can benefit from NuCalm. I know it's done great things for me, at many levels you'll read about in this book. If you're thinking "Hey, this guy is pushing me" and you don't see the value of balance or relaxation, then all I ask is that you read this book before you make up your mind. I intend to keep on spreading the word about NuCalm, so it can help as many people as possible.

By the way, this company is working on different types of physics and different types of outcomes. In fact, I am collaborating with them to develop focused, high-energy "warrior brain" audio files designed to create peak performance brain activity. They are the opposite of the current NuCalm relaxation software files, one of the technology's four parts. In this new project, we want to create exceptional focus and productivity through gamma brain wave function. Be on the lookout for it in the future!

So for all of you who want to create immeasurable differences and achieve a better quality of life, I invite you to learn more about NuCalm. If I can take just 20 to 30 minutes to restore, NuCalm will give me hours of peak performance. I feel stronger, more rested and more focused, and so can you.

Tony Robbins

Life coaching pioneer, author, philanthropist
Palm Beach, Florida
September 2016

PREFACE

If ever there were a born skeptic, it was I. Even as a kid, I had serious reservations about life. There is a photo of me when I was about four years old, looking like a little owl, with my arms folded, and a look on my face that said, "I'm not so sure about this business of growing up and living happily ever after!"

Most kids outgrow their youthful hang-ups, but I didn't. Although I had loving parents, was active in the Boy Scouts, sang in my church choir, played Little League baseball, and did well in school, I continued to take life pretty seriously. At age 10, I did a voice-over for a radio commercial, and soon began modeling clothes and playing small parts in commercials and TV shows. It was fun to get out of school for a few days each month, but, once again, I looked at the glamour around me with a skeptical eye.

By the time I got to college, I was still pretty suspicious about how my life would "work out," and my doubts were immediately confirmed. In my freshman textbook I read the definition of the word "economics." It said that economics is the study of man's attempt to satisfy unlimited desires with limited means. I thought, "I knew it! Even this money business is hopeless by definition!"

After a stint in the Army and graduating from USC Film School, my young life suddenly took a left turn. I became a yoga monk with Self-Realization Fellowship and moved into a California ashram, where I lived for the next 35 years! If I wanted answers to "big picture" questions, surely this was the place to be.

It was an ideal life for an idealist like me. Eventually I took vows as a swami and traveled the world teaching thousands about meditation and mindful living. Yet, unlike the superheroes who conquer the scariest of worldly foes, I soon realized that my main enemy was my own superficial and restless mind! Sitting perfectly still, amidst total silence, during our weekly six-hour meditations, I encountered much about myself that my ego wasn't ready to deal with! But I was sincere, and over the years I spent about 100,000 hours in meditation, coupled with a rigid program of study, introspection and spiritual guidance.

As a counselor to so many people, I learned how challenging it is for the average person to focus the mind—no less reach one's calm center and get in touch with one's unique creativity and intuition. In the monastery, I practiced breathing exercises and yoga postures, and studied the lives of saints. I enjoyed daily group meditations, ate a healthy diet and had the example of monks who had lived a spiritual life for decades. How could a person working two jobs, raising three kids and trying to stay connected to a husband or wife, possibly find the time and energy to cast a personal and professional vision and achieve his or her most meaningful goals?

This is the primary challenge most people face. Today, I am no longer a monk, but I still walk and talk and quack like one! In fact, I'm still doing the same things I did during my monastic years: public speaking, personal counseling, and performing weddings and baptisms.

Every day I work with individuals who are striving to balance their lives, achieve their goals and live fulfilling lives. It requires a lot of maturity and discipline. For many years, I believed that conscious qualities—being present, managing fear, gaining self-confidence, maintaining peak performance and dealing with self-doubt—*could* be achieved by those rare individuals who made a nearly superhuman commitment to self-mastery. But, fortunately, we *all* have some exciting new possibilities.

Some friends introduced me to a neuroscience technology called NuCalm which has enhanced my efforts to relax and center my mind on a daily basis—exactly what I spent decades doing by will power alone.

Our technological age has at last brought us a way to complement our efforts to find inner and outer success, without burning out and making significant compromises in our lives. My NuCalm calms my mind in a matter of minutes, and also clarifies my thinking and gives me greater focus. The result of years of development, it rests on the bedrock of scientific research and has been tested by professionals around the world.

My family uses NuCalm faithfully, and friends who try it are amazed. It doesn't take the place of meditation, but is a way to "jump start" the process of interiorization and rejuvenation. And an added bonus—it produces cumulative results. The more I use it, the greater the benefits I receive.

I can't explain the experience of NuCalm, but I can talk a long time about its benefits. I've never experienced anything quite like this, and I understand different states of consciousness. I am using it every day and find myself becoming more creative and clear, not just less stressed.

I am experiencing a new clarity, which is translating into an avalanche of new creative ideas and actions. I feel like I am seeing life through a more healthy lens. I have greater presence. I have greater clarity and greater clarity leads to confidence. I know more now of who I am, which allows me to be more directly open to what I need to do. My agenda, from being very broad, has moved to very focused!

I don't claim to comprehend the science behind NuCalm. Yet, I'm fascinated by the results. Here's what I know, for sure. Today I'm flying out of Los Angeles for an extended European vacation. Last night I stayed up until 4 a.m., finishing last minute work. With only three hours of sleep, I will use NuCalm this morning, pack my tablet and headset in my carry-on (to use on the long flight to Amsterdam) and I'll arrive tomorrow, without jet lag. Even at my age, I still live a very active life, but now have a way to remain "calmly active and actively calm." I still maintain my daily meditation and mindfulness practices, but my new tool helps me (finally) smile, and even wink, at a whole new world.

Brother Craig Marshall

35-year yoga monk, personal consultant, speaker
Los Angeles, California
September 2016

INTRODUCTION

While I was working with Larry Trivieri on our book *Outstanding Health* in October 2014, my wife Janet told me to try NuCalm and include it in the book "because it really works."

That is no small endorsement. My wife is Janet Hranicky, Ph.D., a clinical psychologist currently working on her medical degree. For more than 25 years, she has been a recognized expert in psychoneuroimmunology and, among her many accomplishments, is co-director of the Comprehensive Cancer Wellness Program at the Hippocrates Health Institute in West Palm Beach, Florida. She learned about the NuCalm technology there, and was impressed with its rapid ability to help cancer patients relax and rest, which helps with healing.

At the time, I decided against her advice because I did not know anything about NuCalm or the people behind it. However now, Larry and I agree enthusiastically with Janet. We decided that NuCalm deserved its own book.

Any technology that can balance the autonomic nervous system is fantastic, because doing so optimizes health. That is what we are all after, and that is what NuCalm does. The proof is in the years of testing and scientific research to qualify for its unique U.S. patent as the only "system or method for balancing and maintaining the health of the human autonomic nervous system."

How NuCalm works, and why the autonomic nervous system is so important to your health, will be explained in detail in this book. Here, I will just mention enough for you to understand why I am so pleased to introduce this exciting technology to you. I would like to share the story of my initial experience with NuCalm, as well as a little about my own background.

A few months after hearing of NuCalm, I had a visit from Jim Poole, CEO of Solace Lifesciences, the company that makes it. He and Janet had been working together with the cancer patients, and they wanted me to examine the technology and the research results. I remember that it was the end of my working day. I was kind of on edge because I had not slept well for two or three weeks. Jim explained everything about the technology, set me up in a comfortable chair and got things going. I could feel the tension reducing in my body, and then I just drifted into a nice, pleasant state. In fact, I was so completely relaxed that I believe I passed out. Jim came back about an hour later to wake me up. That was my introduction to NuCalm.

I loved it. I realized immediately that NuCalm had huge advantages in promoting sleep, reducing stress and giving me an overall sense of well-being. I like to use NuCalm every day. I've got one at home and one at the office. In my busy practice, I actually used to be angry when a patient canceled at the last second. Now, though, I go straight into a NuCalm session. I find that if I can do it regularly, it's extremely beneficial.

It did not take long to realize that NuCalm would help my patients, too. Most of them come from the Los Angeles area and are high-powered, stressed people. I have introduced most of my patients to NuCalm when they complain about stress, explaining how it will benefit them almost immediately. Everybody has loved it, 100 percent of the time. They leave to go about their day looking calm and relaxed. Some have gone on to purchase their own, which I see as a credit to the value that people instantly perceive from using NuCalm.

Believe me, I know something about stress. I started my career as one of the first board-certified emergency room doctors and endured 15 years in Los Angeles ERs before burning out. When a clinic asked me to do nutrition and general practice there, I accepted even though I did not have a clue about nutrition. I remember trying to learn by reading books, going to lectures, listening to tapes, hiring a nutritionist, and doing all these new blood tests...but nobody got any better.

One of the patients who did not get better was my best friend who, I later discovered through blood testing, had mercury toxicity from his silver fillings. I found a referral for a dentist who would replace them, and who was able to pinpoint with an energy medicine device what metals could be put safely into his teeth. His results exactly matched the results of the blood tests I had done. My curiosity led to a discussion with the dentist about his techniques, which in turn led to my 30-year search for the safest, most effective methods to bring my patients to a state of robust health.

I try not to be skeptical about anything, because I think the key to being successful as a doctor is to stay open. I have practiced integrative or holistic medicine, using traditional and alternative techniques, for the past 30 years now. I like to call it "energy medicine."

During these years, my search made plain to me that, philosophically, traditional medicine defines health as the absence of disease. Therefore, if you have normal x-rays, CAT scans, MRIs and blood tests, you are healthy. If you complain, you are either stressed out, need a vacation or you need something to relax.

When people come to me saying, "I don't feel well," they may be speaking of well emotionally, mentally, physically or some combination of the three. You cannot see that "I don't feel well" on an x-ray, a CAT scan or an MRI, and you rarely see it in a blood test. However, on a deep electrical level, you can see imbalances. So, in energy or integrative medicine, we do not refer to diseased organs, we refer to sluggish organs that are not working as efficiently as they should.

From this perspective, we see health as one end of the spectrum and disease as the other. Most people are in the middle. They cannot sleep, they are fatigued, they have allergies, they have bloating, they have distention or they have constipation. They are not diseased, but they are not healthy, either. The holistic doctor says, "How do we get you healthy even though you don't have a disease?" That is a huge difference between the two philosophies.

When they are healthy, people have abundant energy. Health is energy. There is an electrical or energetic level to the body that is the foundation of what my practice has become since beginning my search. That is why I refer to what I do as energy medicine.

Following my conversation with the dentist about my friend, I started my search by taking a course in acupuncture for physicians given by UCLA and a three-year course on energy medicine being taught out of Europe. I realized that I could be much more effective using these kinds of technologies to figure out what people really need, and what dosages are correct. This extended eventually into hormone therapy, as well.

Consequently, I do not have any side effects with the therapies I use, which has been a real boon to my practice. I became popular enough to have patients now from six continents. After Suzanne Somers became a patient, I was pleased to participate in several of her books about health.

Over the years, I have investigated many therapies and technologies, investing in those I think will most help my patients. My office is full of them, and NuCalm is a welcomed addition.

Whenever I get these new technologies, my first thought is "Now how does this help me in my practice?" Of course, the best thought would be "How can I benefit from this myself?" If it helps me, it helps everybody.

I was very open to trying NuCalm in the beginning because I realize that the less stressed I can become, the more effective I can be as a doctor.

Furthermore, I encourage the doctors I know to try NuCalm and see for themselves. Physicians are always looking for ways to help our patients, taking the life or death part of our jobs seriously. I believe that patients cannot help but benefit if the quality of their physician's life improves by reducing stress levels. Everybody benefits down the line. Then I encourage doctors to use NuCalm on their patients because, in the Los Angeles area, there is no shortage of patients complaining about stress.

Although I prefer the word challenges, there are all sorts of stressors that all of us encounter every day, good and bad. These include mental stress like college students studying for finals, emotional stress like arguing with a spouse, nutritional stress like an allergic reaction, environmental stress like pesticide exposure, geopathic stress like electromagnetic fields, and physical stress like injuries.

What is most important to your health is how you respond to stress, and that is governed by the autonomic nervous system. It regulates your next breath, your next heartbeat and your blood pressure, like an automatic or subconscious system. There are two parts to it: the sympathetic, which is your left brain, action-oriented and performance nervous system; and the parasympathetic, which is your right brain, creative, relaxation and regeneration nervous system. If compared to running a hundred-yard dash, your sympathetic would be how fast you can run the race and your parasympathetic would be how long it takes you to get your breath back.

Of the two parts, the parasympathetic is the more important. I use the analogy of the children's song "Row, row, row your boat gently down the stream. Merrily, merrily, merrily, merrily, life is but a dream." You have to get the sympathetic nervous system in gear when you are rowing up stream, when you feel like you have a challenge. The key to life is really to go down stream, to be in the flow. When you have a strong parasympathetic nervous system, you are going down stream. I try to explain to my patients that if you can live feeling as though you are going down stream, you will have a much healthier, happier and more fulfilling life.

The ideal way to be healthy is to have a strong parasympathetic nervous system and to tone down the sympathetic nervous system. We need both, but stress causes an imbalance.

After my introduction to NuCalm, Jim showed me the extensive before and after studies done on cancer patients and athletes. For the research, they would do a heart rate variability test, do a NuCalm session and repeat the test. There was a dramatic reduction in the level of the sympathetic nervous system and an improvement in the parasympathetic nervous system. The best way to see electrical changes in the body is with heart rate variability, so I see NuCalm as a perfect fit with the practice of energy medicine.

Jim's test results were confirmed in my patients who used NuCalm, after testing them with my own heart rate variability machine. I got the same results: the balancing of the autonomic nervous system. I don't need to verify something repeatedly, once or twice and I'm convinced. I could see NuCalm's benefits subjectively, from the effects I was experiencing myself, and objectively, from the test results. That was enough to convince me that this is a great technology.

My patients love NuCalm, too. I've heard comments like, "Wow, I've just landed," or "What an incredible experience," or "I feel so relaxed." After using NuCalm for a half-hour, they are in a little bit of a pleasant, positive altered state, and they don't start verbalizing for the next few minutes. By then I'm on to my next patient, so I don't get to hear much more. My office administrator assures me that we have never had a negative comment.

In my experience, people want to reclaim their power and take care of their own health. To do so, they can eat right, they can exercise, they can take supplements and they can detoxify. All those things are important, but how does one feel well emotionally?

We need to help people feel well emotionally and at the same time strengthen the autonomic nervous system. I think everybody needs to know about anything out there that is non-invasive and easy to do, with quick results to get them healthier. NuCalm is the technology that helps people feel better and healthier, by balancing their autonomic nervous system and keeping it healthy.

That is really what we all want. We all want to feel GREAT.

Michael Galitzer, M.D.

Energy medicine pioneer, author, anti-aging expert
Los Angeles, California
September, 2016

CHAPTER 1

THE PROMISE OF NUCALM

Congratulations! By reading this book, you will discover a revolutionary, patented technology that can shift your body out of *stress* and into a state of profound relaxation—literally within minutes.

We, the authors, have never before seen anything that can so quickly, easily and effectively banish stress while balancing the *autonomic nervous system*, the powerful controller of all other systems in your body.

Allow us to introduce ourselves. Dr. Michael Galitzer is a pioneering integrative physician and clinical expert in anti-aging, regenerative and preventive medicine. Larry Trivieri Jr. is an internationally recognized lay expert and best-selling author in the field of health and wellness. Together we have more than 60 years of combined expertise.

The breakthrough health system we are so excited to introduce to you is NuCalm®. First, allow us to share with you just a few of the many enthusiastic testimonials received from its users:

"I use NuCalm daily because it helps me put all the pieces back together," said Kevin Matthews, a well-known radio personality in Chicago, who is now retired. Kevin suffers from multiple sclerosis and, as is common in people with MS, Kevin reports that he is "fighting my body every day."

As Kevin's condition progressed, he found that the inflammatory response and resultant stress associated with MS were negatively impacting his memory and cognitive function. At times, MS caused his legs "not to work." Then his wife, who dreaded dental appointments like many people, was introduced to the NuCalm technology by her dentist. Astonished by how relaxed she was during her dental procedure—an experience she described as "amazing"—she recommended that Kevin try it as a way to cope better with his MS symptoms. As soon as he did, Kevin also began to experience a significant reduction in stress.

Kevin has continued to use NuCalm on a daily basis. Doing so has helped him regain the full use of his legs, which no longer give out on him due to his illness. Just as importantly, NuCalm is helping Kevin recapture his memories as he writes his autobiography. "I find that using NuCalm restores my past experiences, enabling me to relive them in vivid detail," he said. In addition, his other MS symptoms are now much more manageable than before Kevin began using NuCalm, and his stress levels are greatly reduced.

"NuCalm is my safety net. I rely on it," said Michaela Y., who used the NuCalm technology to resolve four years of high emotional stress. During that time, she had undergone major life changes, including a big move. The resultant stress caused her to suffer from panic attacks and chronically poor sleep.

Only in her 30s, Michaela's physical state was in a downward spiral until she discovered NuCalm. Once she began using it, everything began to improve, even with her ongoing life changes. She sleeps much better and is free of panic attacks. "Today, people ask me all the time how I can be so calm," Michaela said. "The positive difference NuCalm has made in my life is a miracle."

"NuCalm allows me to respond instead of react to stressful situations," said Julie Burns, a registered dietitian and certified clinical nutritionist with a master's in clinical dietetics. She has worked with the Chicago Blackhawks, as well as Chicago's Bears, White Sox and Bulls teams. Burns also consults with individual elite athletes from around the globe, and describes herself as a driven, Type A personality.

Prior to discovering the NuCalm technology, she often lost control in her life by agreeing to too many requests. Ongoing use of NuCalm allows her to "reset," so that she no longer is reactionary to stressful situations. Now, Burns feels more in control of her life, and can decline requests that detract from her focus and goals.

Once she personally experienced the benefits that NuCalm offers, Burns worked with the training staff of the Blackhawks to encourage the players to use NuCalm.

Beginning in 2012, the entire Blackhawks team began using NuCalm regularly. Since then, they have won the Stanley Cup championship twice, including their 4-2 game victory over the Tampa Lightning in 2015. According to the Blackhawks' medical staff, the NuCalm technology was one of the keys to the players' success. Head trainer Mike Gapski said it was the most difficult championship of the three Stanley Cup titles the team has won since 2010. "Every playoff game was intense and they just kept getting tougher and tougher," he said, adding, "The crucial part of this game is recovery. NuCalm played an important role for us, especially during the playoffs."

Sports performance is only one area where NuCalm is making an impressive impact. As mentioned earlier, dentists use the NuCalm technology with significant, positive effects. Experts at the Dental Fears Research Clinic of the University of Washington say that "up to 75 percent of adults have at least some anxiety about going to the dentist,"[1] and perhaps 20 percent experience enough anxiety that they go to the dentist "only when absolutely necessary."[2] NuCalm offers a proven solution, changing their dental experience from one of anxiety and discomfort to one that is relaxing and refreshing.

More than 700,000 dental patients across five continents have experienced the NuCalm technology during visits to their dentists. Of all NuCalm patients surveyed afterward, 95 percent say they would use it again and 98 percent would recommend NuCalm to family and friends. Here is a sampling of actual comments from some of the patients who were surveyed:

"I feel completely relaxed. If it worked on me it will work on anyone."

"I have a euphoric sense. I forgot a dental procedure was being done."

"I am always a big chicken in the chair. Now I feel like I can do anything with NuCalm."

"I could not have ever made it through my appointment without

NuCalm. In fact, I ran out of my dentist's office before my appointment started last time."

"I can't really explain it. I just feel really good. Thank you."

"I will never have another health care procedure done without NuCalm."

"NuCalm was a very relaxing, therapeutic experience. I have chronic neck and shoulder pain. After NuCalm I had no pain, which is remarkable. Can I have this done every month?"

Dentists who use the NuCalm technology in their practice are just as excited and relieved as their patients by the results NuCalm produces. Here are some of their comments:

"Three days after using NuCalm, it hit me. I was driving to work when I realized that after 28 years of practicing dentistry, I would no longer have to swallow all of my patients' fear and anxiety. The realization brought me to tears! Now after two weeks of using this amazing technique, my team and I can't wait to get the next patient started. It takes us less than three minutes to get the patient started, then another three to five minutes before the patient is completely relaxed, and I can begin their dental procedure. Our patients are calm, still and relaxed throughout the entire appointment, and when it is over they thank us for a great experience...at the dentist! How cool is that? NuCalm is making me a hero with my patients and at the end of the day I go home refreshed and not tired! It is a whole new ballgame and I look forward to getting back to the office each morning and turning the next patient on to NuCalm!" **Dr. Peter T. Harnois, D.D.S., president of the Illinois Academy of Facial Esthetics, Chicago, Illinois.**

"We have treated in excess of 1,000 patients in our practice using this technology. In fact, if it were taken away from our practice today, we feel we would be doing our patients a disservice. Having a system today that helps remove the anxiety factor from the dental equation makes absolute sense. Everyone benefits. Using NuCalm today is certainly a win-win for our patients, our teams and ourselves. What a great system! The bonus of course is, if we are stressed or anxious, we can always NuCalm ourselves." **Dr. Mervyn Druian, B.D.S (RAND) D.G.D.P RCS, London, UK.**

"For myself, this technology has allowed me to be more efficient. I have cut my procedure times down by 30 to 40 percent in most cases. I am less stressed because my patients are at ease. The system is easy to use and within three minutes our patients are hooked up and relaxing. The fact that I can still communicate with them, and they can respond as necessary, makes my job that much easier. I leave my office feeling more relaxed. I never realized how much stress is transferred to me and my team just from patient encounters. We become anesthetized to it, but once I see my patient relax then I become more relaxed. Patients are referring family members and friends that have feared going to the dentist for years. It's amazing to witness our patients' sense of tranquility. When we see our patients in a state of pleasure rather than in a state of apprehension, it is overwhelming to me and my team." **Dr. Louis Kaufman, D.D.S., Chicago, Illinois.**

Summing up the views of fellow dentists who now employ the NuCalm technology in their practices, Dr. Omer Reed, a dental surgeon from Phoenix, Arizona, said, "Rarely does a solution this profound get launched into the dental industry. NuCalm is going to change dentistry."

Based on what you have read so far, you can understand why we are so excited about sharing NuCalm with you. It is the only patented technology in the world for balancing and maintaining the health of the human autonomic nervous system.

In the pages ahead, you will learn how and why NuCalm works. You will meet NuCalm's inventor, Dr. G. Blake Holloway, and discover how he came to develop NuCalm by scientifically sequencing and combining four all-natural, drug-free relaxation therapies into one overall system. You will see how this system closely and elegantly mimics your body's own physiological processes for dealing with stress and preparing for deep relaxation.

In addition, you will discover the numerous and immediate health benefits that NuCalm provides. These include:

- Reducing stress
- Inhibiting unnecessary production of stress hormones
- Calming nerves
- Improving sleep quality
- Helping reverse sleep disorders such as insomnia
- Enhancing immune function
- Enhancing overall heart health and cardiovascular function
- Improving respiratory health and sinus conditions
- Providing pain relief
- Relieving anxiety and fears
- Restoring the body's biological clock and circadian rhythms
- Speeding recovery from physical exertion and injury.

Moreover, you will discover the many health conditions for which the NuCalm technology is proving to be beneficial, ranging from dental problems to cancer, heart disease and post-traumatic stress disorder (PTSD).

NuCalm provides a multitude of other benefits, making it the therapy of choice for elite athletes, business executives, creative artists and many others who are concerned with optimal performance in their daily lives. As you will learn, this technology can significantly enhance focus, concentration and mental alertness, while simultaneously increasing creativity and problem-solving skills. NuCalm literally puts you "in the zone" on demand.

To fully appreciate how and why NuCalm is capable of providing such a wide range of benefits, however, you first need to understand more about the most significant saboteur that you face in your daily life: *stress.*

To discover how this culprit can drain your ability to function efficiently and happily, please continue to Chapter 2.

Chapter 2

Stress: The Great Saboteur

Stress, more than anything else, has the greatest potential to sabotage every aspect of your life: your health, your relationships, your work, your productivity, your brain function and cognitive abilities, and even your ability to simply enjoy your day. Yet despite all we know about the importance of managing stress, as a society we are significantly stressed out.

This is confirmed by the *2015 Stress in America* survey conducted by the American Psychological Association. According to the "Stress Snapshot" published on the APA's website:

- Compared to the previous year, 34 percent of adults reported that their stress had increased.[1]

- Even worse, on a scale of 1 (little to no stress) to 10 (extremely high stress), 24 percent of all Americans reported their stress level at 8 or above. This compared to 18 percent in 2014, and was the highest percentage of extreme stress reported since 2010.[2]

- Nearly a third (31 percent) of Americans reported that stress had a strong or very strong negative impact on their physical health, and 32 percent reported the same with regard to their mental and emotional health. These were up significantly from 2014 levels of 25 and 28 percent, respectively.[3]

Respondents reported that, in the month before the survey, their stress-related symptoms included: nervousness or anxiety (42 percent), depression or sadness (37 percent), constant worry (33 percent), irritability or anger (37 percent), overeating (39 percent), lying awake at night (46 percent), impatience or yelling at a spouse (47 percent), impatience with co-workers (25 percent), and overwhelm (25 percent).[4]

While a large number (63 percent) of Americans felt they were doing enough to manage stress, actually engaging in stress management activities was infrequent (49 percent) or not at all (18 percent).[5] Although not asked in the 2015 APA stress survey, participants in APA's 2012 survey reported that the primary obstacles to stress management activities were:

- lack of willpower (31 percent)

- lack of time (22 percent)

- cost to make needed changes (16 percent)

- stress itself (12 percent).[6]

Given the above statistics, we clearly need a more effective solution to stress.

Stress and Your Health

Chronic stress, quite simply, threatens your health and longevity. According to the American Institute of Stress, "it's hard to think of any disease in which stress cannot play an aggravating role or any part of the body that is not affected...(and) this list will undoubtedly grow as the extensive ramifications of stress are increasingly being appreciated.[7]

Even research reported in the conservative *Journal of the American Medical Association* states, "Exposures to chronic stress are considered the most toxic because they are most likely to result in long-term or permanent changes in the emotional, physiological, and behavioral responses that influence susceptibility to and (the) course of disease."[8]

A landmark 20-year study of British civil servants, called the Whitehall Study, was conducted by researchers at the University of London beginning in 1967. It forever changed the discourse about causes of heart disease, introducing stress as a contributing factor. By

2008, the continuing Whitehall research had defined the mechanisms linking stress to coronary heart disease.[9]

In the U.S., statistical reports indicate that the toll of heart disease and cancer is enormous, together accounting for more than 3,500 deaths per day.

According to the American Cancer Society's report, *Cancer Facts and Figures 2015*, "About 1,658,370 new cancer cases are expected to be diagnosed in 2015. This estimate does not include carcinoma in situ (noninvasive cancer) of any site except urinary bladder, nor does it include basal cell or squamous cell skin cancers, which are not required to be reported to cancer registries... In 2015, about 589,430 Americans (were) expected to die of cancer, or about 1,620 people per day. Cancer is the second most common cause of death in the US, exceeded only by heart disease, and accounts for nearly 1 of every 4 deaths."[10]

As noted above, the incidence of heart disease in the U.S., and the combined number of deaths from heart attacks and stroke, is an even greater threat than cancer. More than 85 million Americans are living with heart disease or the aftereffects of stroke,[11] and each year heart disease and stroke combine to kill nearly 787,000 people,[12] according to the *2015 Heart Disease and Stroke Statistics Update* compiled by the American Heart Association, the CDC, the National Institutes of Health and other government agencies. That equals 2,150 deaths each day, or one death every 40 seconds.[13] Heart disease is also the No. 1 killer of women in the U.S., causing them about the same number of deaths each year as cancer, chronic lower respiratory diseases and diabetes combined.[14]

A growing number of researchers point out that improving stress management skills, along with making healthier lifestyle choices, could significantly reduce these numbers.

However, despite the compelling scientific evidence linking stress to illness, doctors usually give little attention to managing stress when they consult with their patients. Although doctors may advise their patients to try to relax more, rarely do they provide effective self-care tools for doing so. Tranquilizing drugs may offer temporary relief, but they do not address the underlying problem and often have negative side effects.

How Stress Leads to Disease

All of us are exposed to stress every day. Without stress, life as we know it would not be possible. Certain types of stress are essential for good health.

For example, when you exercise your muscles, you are placing them under stress. This type of stress is a positive thing, because it strengthens and builds your muscles and keeps your body in a growth mode. Stress also plays a health-supporting role in stretching and aerobic exercises, which result in a stronger abdominal core and greater flexibility. Your body responds to these positive stresses as a healthy challenge.

In short, your body is designed not only to cope with a certain amount of stress, but actually to depend on some level of stress for its survival.

Negative stress, on the other hand, is rightly perceived by your body as a threat. When negative stress is present, your body shifts into a defensive mode. As long as you are in defense mode, you cannot grow further.

How the body perceives stress provides a clue to when stress causes disease. After spending decades investigating how and why stress causes illness, former Stanford biologist Bruce Lipton, Ph.D., coined the phrase "New Biology"[15] to counter the fatalistic philosophy in current medicine that illness is primarily a matter of fate, shaped by one's genes. He believes that although we may be born with genetic predispositions toward certain types of illnesses, it is our habitual thoughts and beliefs, along with environmental factors, that have the most influence over whether we get sick. Scientists and physicians in our health care system are moving toward his view that emotions can influence illness.

To better understand how thoughts and beliefs can impact your health, let's take a closer look at how the body is designed to protect itself from disease. No doubt, you are familiar with the immune system. Doctors and patients alike consider the immune system to be the human body's first line of defense against disease. Its task is to identify invading microorganisms (bacteria, fungi, parasites and viruses) and to attack and eliminate them before they can cause harm to the body's cells, tissues and organs.

The common cold is an example of how stress and its negative thoughts affect the immune system, and therefore your health. Colds are said to be caused by a class of virus known as rhinoviruses. However, the virus itself actually does not cause a cold. If that were the case, then everyone exposed to rhinoviruses would automatically catch a cold. Yet many people, such as doctors and nurses, are not affected and do not develop colds, despite even prolonged exposure.

The reason these people remain healthy is simple: they have adaptable and resilient immune systems that are able to ward off the cold virus.[16] In other words, their immune systems are not in a state of stress.

As you can see, it is not the cold virus, but your immune system's ability to function optimally that determines if you will develop a cold. Therefore, to protect yourself against a cold, as well as many potential disease conditions, your best precaution is to maintain your immune system in a healthy state. This includes not only eating right, exercising and getting adequate amounts of restorative sleep, but also effectively managing stress in all of its forms (physical, mental, emotional, spiritual, social, etc.).

As important as the immune system is to good health, there is another system within the body that is equally, and perhaps even more, important. This is the *hypothalamic-pituitary-adrenal axis*, called the HPA axis, which is a key part of the hormonal system.

The purpose of the HPA axis is to spring into action at the first sign of any external threats to the body. With no threats, the HPA axis is in what might be described as idle mode. This allows the rest of your body to flourish the way that nature intended. However, when the *hypothalamus* center in the brain perceives an outside threat, it signals the HPA axis to do its job. This is the fight-or-flight response.

As soon as this signal is given, your body's adrenal glands increase production of cortisol, adrenaline and other stress hormones, releasing them into the blood stream. Once this happens, blood vessels that supply oxygen and nutrients to your cells and organs are constricted so that more blood can flow to tissues in your extremities. Necessarily, when you see a threat, you must quickly use your arms and legs to fend off external attacks or get out of harm's way.

Prior to this response, the blood in the body is concentrated in the abdominal visceral organs: the adrenal glands, kidneys, liver, gall bladder, stomach, intestines, colon and appendix. These organs are responsible for digestion and absorption of food and nutrients, for excretion, and for various other functions that provide proper cell growth and production of cellular energy. As blood rushes to the tissues of the arms and legs, the visceral organs cannot function at 100 percent, causing all growth-related activities in the body to be limited. As you can imagine, if this response continues for sustained periods, all of those activities will start to suffer.

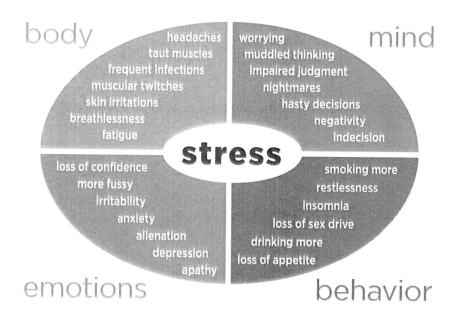

In our ancient past, the *fight-or-flight* response played an essential role in helping our ancestors stay alive in the face of dangers such as attacking animals and threats such as earthquakes, floods and volcanic eruptions. Today, most of us do not face these types of physical dangers; and even when we do, they usually are short-lived.

Interestingly, actual physical danger is not necessary to trigger the fight-or-flight response.[17] Your thoughts and beliefs can trigger it, too. Simply put, if you habitually focus on limiting or negative thoughts and beliefs, your body can behave as if it is in danger. Although the adrenaline rush caused by an actual physical threat usually doesn't occur, the other aspects of the fight-or-flight response still take place and, moreover, persist for long periods. This results in the chronic production of stress hormones.

Chronically elevated stress hormones cause a chronically suppressed immune function, leading to a greater susceptibility to infectious disease. Furthermore, because of how chronic stress negatively impacts the visceral organs, many bodily functions also are suppressed, setting the stage for impaired digestion, increased muscle tension, and eventual declines in cell and tissue functions.

Now you can understand how stress is a major health risk factor, not only for heart disease and for cancer, but for gastrointestinal disorders, skin problems, neurological and emotional disorders, and a range of conditions related to immune dysfunction including the common cold, arthritis, herpes and even AIDS. Additionally, chronic stress in middle age can play a role decades later in the onset of Alzheimer's disease and dementia,[18] most likely because of how chronic stress increases certain hormones that negatively affect the brain.

Sleep disorders are another stress-related problem. To achieve healthy sleep, the normal cycle of hormone production, especially cortisol, must operate efficiently. When you are healthy, cortisol levels are highest in the morning (6-8 a.m.) and lowest in the evening, when they continue at a low level as you fall asleep. This allows your body to release sleep-enhancing hormones, such as melatonin and serotonin, leading to deep, restful sleep.

Stress interferes with this process. When we are stressed, cortisol levels remain high, even into the night, and prevent restful sleep. Over time, the cycle of cortisol production becomes unbalanced. The cycle can even reverse, with cortisol levels spiking in the evening and falling in the morning, resulting in feelings of exhaustion. Insomnia and intermittent sleep are both common examples of sleep disorders associated with nighttime spikes in cortisol and other stress hormones, which can include adrenaline.[19]

Moreover, stress compromises the amount and quality of restorative sleep, the only time your cells can remove toxins and repair themselves. As you can imagine, prolonged lack of restorative sleep decreases your cellular health and increases your risk of disease.[20]

Stress also plays a significant role in the onset of anxiety and depression because of how it affects the brain and the nervous system.[21] According to the National Institute of Mental Health, anxiety disorders are the most common type of mental illness in the U.S., affecting approximately 40 million Americans of age 18 years and older (18 percent of the adult population).[22] Estimates are that at least 17 percent of the U.S. population will suffer from serious depression at some point.[23] Nearly half of Americans diagnosed with depression also are afflicted with an anxiety disorder.[24]

Based on these statistics, it is not surprising that antidepressant and anti-anxiety medications are among the top classes of drugs sold in the U.S. Some years, they account for more than 250 million prescriptions.[25] Bear in mind, the entire U.S. population is approximately 321 million people.

Given the steady increase of antidepressant drug use,[26] a growing number of health experts warn that we could become addicted to some such drugs,[27] all of which are fraught with the risk for serious side effects.[28]

Consider for a moment issues beyond health questions. How much do Americans spend on these and other drugs prescribed for stress-related problems? If they could save even a portion of this expense through more natural stress management, how would that help them?

Similarly, could our nation's economy improve through a decrease in stress-related problems? Consider that the U.S. workforce suffers seriously from the effects of stress, as shown by these statistics:[29]

- An average of one million U.S. employees miss work every day due to stress-related disorders, costing employers some $602 per employee each year

- As much as 80 percent of all industrial accidents are due to stress

- Some 60 percent of workers report losing productivity due to stress

- Of all visits to primary care physicians in the U.S., up to 90 percent are directly due to stress-related complaints.

As we will discuss in more detail, by reducing stress and improving the brain's ability to cope with it, all of these alarming numbers could be reduced significantly.

Based on the above explanations, it is clear that dealing with stress effectively is one of the most important steps you can take to ensure your health. As you will discover in the rest of this book, regular use of NuCalm is a powerful way to do just that.

Potential Sources of Stress in Your Life

There are various types of stress and each of them has associated triggers. The most common types of stress and their triggers are:

Physical stress

Causes include allergens, temperature extremes, physical pain or trauma, physical inactivity, overexertion, illness and lack of restorative sleep.

Emotional stress

Causes include divorce or other breakups, death, suffering or chronic illness in yourself or your loved ones, lack of nurturing relationships or friends, unresolved life issues from the past, and suppressed or inappropriately expressed emotions such as anger, anxiety, depression, fear and guilt.

Social stress

Causes include politics, job promotions or demotions, financial issues, and relationship issues with a spouse or significant other, family members, friends, co-workers or unpleasant neighbors.

Environmental stress

Causes include exposure to fluorescent lights, computers and computer printers, cell phones, household appliances, allergens, chemicals and other environmental toxins.

Spiritual stress

Causes include not knowing your life's purpose, fear of death and/ or the afterlife, lack of faith, and a variety of other existential issues, all of which can cause or worsen a spiritual crisis.

Distorted Thinking Patterns

Often it is not the events in your life that cause stress, it is how you react to them. Most events, by themselves, are neutral.

For example, although nobody likes being stuck in traffic, that doesn't mean a traffic jam needs to be stressful. Common reactions are stress producing—such as anger, frustration, impatience and tension—but many people react calmly to traffic jams. Some even recognize them as an opportunity to devote time to something constructive, such as planning activities for later in the day.

Based on the above example, you can understand that how people react to potential stressors is largely due to how they think about them. Many stressors are not stressors at all, including traffic jams. How you think about a neutral event determines if it will cause stress in your life.

Thoughts that cause stress are usually what psychologists refer to as distorted thinking. We distort things when we don't see them as they are, but as we think they are. Continuing with the example above, a traffic jam is neither good nor bad. It has no power over you beyond slowing your arrival at your destination. If you think a traffic jam is a reason to become stressed and upset, then that is exactly what you most likely will feel the next time you find yourself stuck in traffic. However, if you think traffic jams are just minor inconveniences, then it is very likely that you won't be stressed when you experience one.

Here are two other common examples of how distorted thinking and stress can combine to negatively impact your life. First, consider a man who can't find his car keys when he's about to leave for an important meeting, with much riding on its outcome. As he searches, the thought of being late for the meeting takes hold of him, causing a surge of stress hormones to flood through his body. The hormones make his heart race, his blood pressure rise and his breathing constrict. He may start to panic or become angry as his search continues. He may even blame his wife or children for losing his keys. After 15 minutes of running around and stressing more and more, he suddenly finds the keys in the pocket of the coat he has been wearing all along.

Had he been able to remain calm and resist panic, he most likely would have discovered his keys quickly and been on his way. Distorted thinking and the stress it triggered combined to prevent him from finding his keys. He wasted precious time and, in all likelihood, was late for his meeting, exactly as he had feared. Moreover, the flood of stress hormones continued to take a toll on his body long after he found his keys.

In the next example, imagine the same man stressing about another work-related issue, one that he feels pressured to resolve. He is unable to find a solution and obsesses over the problem. His small child, in the same room, seeks attention by repeatedly calling out, "Daddy," only to be ignored. When at last he notices his child, the man realizes how his stress and agitated thoughts distracted him from one of the most important people in his world.

By recognizing the role thoughts play in determining your reactions, you can understand why consciously choosing your thoughts makes a difference in how much stress affects you. You can see how stress upsets your emotional balance and clouds your ability to think clearly. As we will explain, regular use of the NuCalm technology offers tremendous benefit in this area.

The Stressed Autonomic Nervous System

Your body has a variety of regulatory processes designed to maintain good energy flow and which act together to maintain *homeostasis,* or stability and balance in the body's functions. Efficient regulation controls the ability of an organ or tissue to respond appropriately to a stimulus, which is a cardinal feature of optimal health.

The system in your body that has the fastest and most profound effect on regulation is the autonomic nervous system. It makes adjustments within seconds and interacts with the slower endocrine (hormone) system, which takes from minutes to hours to develop effects.

The main link between the body's nervous systems and its endocrine system is the hypothalamus, a small gland in the brain. It acts as the hormone control center, similar to the thermostat in your home. The brain sends messages to the hypothalamus, which releases hormonal messages to its neighbor, the pituitary gland. In response, the pituitary gland produces hormones that in turn stimulate target glands—such as the adrenals, thyroid, ovaries and testes—to produce their hormones.

Also involved in the process of regulation are the lymphatic system and the intestines, both small and large, as well as the healthy intestinal flora they contain. They work both to ensure that your body efficiently assimilates nutrients from food, and to aid in elimination of internal and external toxins. They also play essential roles in maintaining and regulating your immune system.

The importance of the autonomic nervous system to regulation merits further explanation.

Sometimes called the automatic or subconscious nervous system, the autonomic nervous system controls heart activity by lowering or raising the pulse rate. It also controls blood pressure, breathing, intestinal activity, temperature regulation and many other functions. It is in direct contact with both the central nervous system (brain and spinal cord) and the peripheral nervous system (motor and sensory nerves).

Because it controls all these and other mechanisms of regulation, and thus your body's ability to react and adapt to stressors and changes, the autonomic nervous system has great importance to your health. Imagine it as an information transfer system. If you think of the brain as the central power station, the autonomic nervous system is like the power cables leading to all the buildings.

The autonomic nervous system has two integrated parts—the *sympathetic nervous system* and the *parasympathetic nervous system*. The sympathetic nervous system is more active during the day and is responsible for both energy production and your body's stress-coping mechanisms. These mechanisms include fight-or-flight responses and immune stimulation, each triggered by emergencies. The parasympathetic system, by contrast, is more active at night and is engaged in energy recovery, repair, regeneration and relaxation.

Overall, the sympathetic system is related to performance and the parasympathetic system oversees recovery. Both are important. In sports, for example, we may be more concerned with an athlete's performance—how fast he can run a 100-yard dash—than with how long it takes him to catch his breath. Yet it is often the second issue that best determines overall athletic condition and achievement. Thus, the stronger your parasympathetic nervous system, the healthier you will be, because you will be able to perform well without an excessive expenditure of energy.

Many people unknowingly go through life with their sympathetic nervous system in overdrive and with insufficient parasympathetic activity, resulting in chronic states of physical stress and diminished health. For example, the sympathetic nervous system controls the level of tension in muscles. Frequently, it is overactive and out of balance in relation to the parasympathetic system. This imbalance can lead to muscle problems such as tension, fatigue and spasm.

The health of your heart and cardiovascular system are especially dependent on balanced functioning between the sympathetic and parasympathetic nervous systems. As research into heart disease continues to progress, it appears that the underlying causes of heart disease, including heart attacks, can be traced to the autonomic nervous system. Understanding its link to heart disease is leading to a revolution in treatment and prevention.[30]

When it comes to reversing and preventing heart disease, the parasympathetic nervous system is particularly important. It uses the *vagus nerve* to send impulses to the heart. The vagus nerve, under the direction of the parasympathetic nervous system, slows and relaxes the heart. By contrast, the sympathetic nervous system causes the heart to beat faster, especially when it activates the fight-or-flight response.

Heart Rate Variability

The overall functioning of the autonomic nervous system can be assessed very easily with an in-office test for heart rate variability (HRV). During this test, a sensor attached to the chest area records the heartbeat for two minutes while the patient is lying down, and for another two minutes while the patient stands. The results are plotted or graphed to reveal the activity of the sympathetic and parasympathetic nervous systems, with values ranging between +4 and -4 for each.

HRV refers to differences in the length of each heartbeat. You might conclude that in a person with a pulse of 60 beats per minute, each beat would last one second. If that were so, however, there would be no heart rate variability, a definite symptom of chronic disease.

On the other hand, if one beat lasting 1.0 second is immediately followed by a beat of .98 seconds, followed by the next beat of 1.02 seconds, followed by the next beat of .97 seconds, this would indicate excellent heart rate variability. The patient would be considered quite healthy, with a positive reading on the parasympathetic nervous system.

A decrease in, or lack of, heart rate variability is a common risk factor for many chronic diseases.[33] We will cover HRV testing and its importance as an effective diagnostic tool in Chapter 4.

According to Thomas Cowan, M.D., who has spent years researching the link between diminished parasympathetic activity and heart disease, "...an imbalance in these two branches (sympathetic and parasympathetic) is responsible for the vast majority of heart disease."[31]

Studies in Germany showed that patients with ischemic heart disease can have a reduction in parasympathetic activity of 33 percent or more, and that some 80 percent of myocardial ischemic events are triggered by "drastic decreases in cardiac vagal (parasympathetic) activity."[32] Ischemia is characterized by restricted blood flow to the heart and its tissues, which could cause a loss of oxygen and reduce energy supply.

Researchers are able to conduct these studies using a diagnostic test, called *heart rate variability*, to accurately measure both sympathetic and parasympathetic activity in real time.

Coming from the opposite direction, subjects with healthy para-sympathetic activity did not suffer from ischemic events when they experienced spikes in their sympathetic activity due to physical or emotional shocks.[34] The significance of this research is that increased activation of the sympathetic nervous system does not seem to cause heart attacks and other types of heart disease, unless such activation is preceded by decreased parasympathetic activity.

"We are meant to have times of excess sympathetic activity; that is normal life. What's dangerous to our health is the ongoing, persistent decrease in our parasympathetic, or life-restoring, activity," Dr. Cowan said.

Based on this new understanding of heart disease, researchers are beginning to see that heart attacks and other types of heart disease may not occur unless there is first a decrease in parasympathetic activity. In a typical disease scenario, this decrease is followed by an increase in sympathetic activity, usually due to a fight-or-flight response to physical, emotional or other stressors. This combination of events results in heart cells dramatically increasing their production of lactic acid, which occurs in virtually 100 percent of heart attack events,[35] whether or not the coronary arteries are negatively impacted.

The increased acidity makes heart cell walls rigid and less able to contract,[36] leading to edema (swelling) and impaired function of the heart muscle itself, as well as to heart cell death. All of these conditions contribute to causing heart attacks. Furthermore, the swelling of heart tissue changes pressure in the arteries that run through the affected area of the heart. The increase in pressure, in turn, causes vulnerable plaque in the arteries to rupture, further blocking the arteries involved and/or creating dangerous clots.

Most important to remember is that none of it happens unless and until parasympathetic activity first decreases. "Only this explanation accounts for all of the observable phenomena associated with heart disease," Dr. Cowan said. "The true origin of heart disease could not be more clear."

Decreased parasympathetic activity caused by stress and the ensuing cascade of events in the heart negatively affect the endothelium,[37,38] which is the very thin layer of cells that line your body's arteries. A healthy endothelium is necessary for proper blood flow and overall cardiovascular function, especially in the smooth vascular muscle that makes up most of the blood vessel walls.

These negative effects on the endothelium all are linked to heart disease. The three possible negative reactions are inflammation, oxidative stress or increased levels of free radicals, and vascular autoimmune dysfunction, in which the body mistakenly attacks its own blood vessels with antibodies.

Compounding this problem, each time blood vessels and the endothelium are negatively affected they create a type of memory, which can trigger heightened reactions to subsequent incidents. This is true even if the subsequent harm is seemingly of little consequence. Research[39,40,41] has shown, for instance, that even short-term exposure to an inflammatory agent, such as sugar, can lead to a long-term inflammatory response and/or damage in blood vessels and tissue.

Important to emphasize is that problems within the heart and overall cardiovascular system most often occur only if there is first a decrease in parasympathetic activity. For example, atherosclerosis is a result of endothelial dysfunction and is viewed as a significant risk factor for heart disease. Having atherosclerosis does not mean that angina, heart attack or other types of heart disease will occur. So long as parasympathetic activity is healthy, the autonomic functions may slow development of atherosclerosis or even prevent acute coronary syndrome.[42]

This does not mean that you can, or should, ignore atherosclerosis if it is present, any more than you should ignore any other risk factors linked to heart disease. All such factors need to be addressed.

A healthy parasympathetic nervous system, however, is of paramount importance when it comes to protecting your heart. NuCalm's ability to balance and improve parasympathetic nervous system activity offers a groundbreaking method for helping reduce the risk and incidence of our nation's No.1 killer, and many other unhealthy conditions, as we will explore in Chapter 5.

Common Ways of Dealing with Stress

Given how rampant stress is in our society, more and more people are seeking ways to cope with their stress levels. What follows is a brief overview of some of the most common approaches to stress management.

Stress Medications

As mentioned above, the use of pharmaceutical drugs, including antidepressants and anti-anxiety medications, is widespread in our society. Although such medications have their place, they carry the risk for a variety of potentially harmful side effects, and should be used only under strict supervision. Reliance on such drugs can be expensive, even with health insurance, and may require regular medical check-ups. These drugs can help relieve stress symptoms, but they do not address the underlying causes of stress.

Nutrient Supplementation and Diet

Nutritional deficiencies, along with poor diet, can cause stress and worsen symptoms of anxiety, depression and hyperactivity, which in turn create more feelings of stress and set a vicious cycle in motion.

To help avoid nutritional deficiencies and combat stress, you first need to address your eating habits. Ideally, your diet needs to be free of all foods to which you may be allergic or sensitive, and free of food additives, sugar, sodas and simple carbohydrates. Drink plenty of pure, filtered water throughout the day, and minimize your alcohol intake to no more than one glass of red wine or beer per day. You should limit your caffeine intake, since too much can overstimulate and leave you more susceptible to stress. Skipping breakfast adds to stress levels by making you more tired and irritable.

Certain nutrients improve resistance to stress, restore feelings of calm and relaxation, and promote restful sleep. Among these are the B vitamin inositol (B8), the mineral magnesium, and the amino acids *GABA (gamma amino butyric acid)*, glycine, taurine, L-Theanine and N-Acetyl-L-Tyrosine.

Two other nutritional supplements effective for stress relief and restful sleep are Lactium® and Phenibut (4-Amino-3Phenyl-Butyric Acid). Lactium is a natural substance derived from milk proteins and peptides. Clinical research has shown that Lactium significantly improves a variety of factors related to sleep disorders, including insomnia.[43] Multiple published clinical studies also have shown Lactium to be safe and effective for regulating the major effects of stress, including blood pressure and heart rate recovery.[44,45]

Phenibut is a derivative of GABA, with an added phenyl ring, which enables it to cross the blood-brain barrier. Phenibut was discovered by Russian scientists in the 1960s, and is widely used in Russia as a treatment for anxiety, insomnia and other sleep disorders, and for various stress conditions including PTSD. Research also suggests that Phenibut may act as a nootropic, which means it can enhance neurological functions such as learning, cognition and memory.[47]

All of the above ingredients are included in NuCalm's proprietary nutritional formula, one of its four components detailed in Chapter 3.

Exercise

Physical exercise is another effective means of reducing stress, so long as you do not overdo it. Unfortunately, many people fail to get even a minimal amount of exercise on a regular basis, including something as simple as going for a walk. As a nation, we have become increasingly sedentary. The most common excuse used by people who do not exercise is that they do not have time. Other common challenges to regular exercise include pre-existing medical conditions or lack of knowledge about how to get started.

Meditation

Meditation is perhaps the world's oldest method for dealing with stress, and provides a wealth of other significant benefits. Meditation has been an integral part of spiritual disciplines in both the East and West for thousands of years.

Since the 1960s, western scientists have extensively researched meditation practices. A large body of research has found that meditation, when practiced once or twice a day, results in numerous physical and psychological benefits. These studies showed it reduces many of the physiological and biochemical markers associated with stress, through decreased heart rate, decreased respiration rate and improved regulation of stress hormones such as cortisol.[47] In addition, regular meditation increased brain wave activity associated with relaxation.

Meditation can be defined as any activity that keeps your attention pleasantly anchored in the present moment. In this state, your mind becomes calm and focused, and less apt to react to memories of the past or concerns about the future. Such reactions are major sources of chronic stress and can negatively affect your health.

The simplest form of meditation involves sitting quietly and focusing your attention on your breath. When you are stressed, anxious, agitated, distracted, frightened or otherwise upset, your breathing rate will tend to be shallow, rapid or uneven. When your mind is calm and focused, your breath becomes slow, deep and regular. Daily practice of meditation leads to improved respiration rates, which in turn provide the health benefits described previously.

Research has shown that the more people meditate, the more resistant they become to reactive behaviors and thought patterns that can cause stress and impair health. Long-term practitioners of meditation also tend to be calmer, happier and more energetic than they were before learning to meditate.[48,49]

Yet, one of the principle drawbacks of meditation is that it takes daily practice and time—often months and even years—before its benefits truly begin to manifest. When we are stressed out and want immediate relief, time is not something we can afford to spend.

Yoga and Tai Chi

Two health practices that incorporate both exercise and the breathing aspects of meditation are yoga and tai chi. Both have grown in popularity in the U.S. over the past few decades. Numerous studies confirm that regular practice of either one can provide a wide range of health benefits, including stress relief. [50,51]

However, as with meditation and other forms of exercise, the benefits of yoga and tai chi take time to accrue and become noticeable. Moreover, training under a skilled practitioner is necessary to perform yoga or tai chi effectively, requiring time and expense. Such practitioners are not available in all areas of the U.S.

Alcohol and Illegal Drugs

Sadly, abuse of alcohol and the use of illegal drugs are still widely prevalent ways that many people seek relief from stress and other problems. Both can damage or worsen health, and destroy lives and families. Alcohol abuse alone results in more than 100,000 deaths in the U.S. each year, ranging from disease to traffic fatalities.[52] Alcohol is the most commonly abused substance by children and teens[53] and nearly one-third of young drivers killed in crashes had been drinking.[54] Clearly, substance abuse is not the answer for stress relief or any other life problems.

An Easier, Elegant Solution to Stress

With the exception of alcohol and drug abuse, of course, all of the above stress management options offer proven benefits for stress-related issues. As noted, however, all of those remaining, except nutritional supplementation, can be challenging and slow at producing the results that stress-harried people are seeking. Still, all of the positive options have their place and we certainly recommend them.

Imagine for a moment, though, being able to achieve all of the mentioned benefits and more, yet do so quickly and without effort--with no need to go anywhere, no need to be trained and no need for medical supervision.

Now imagine something even better: a solution to stress that goes even deeper and requires less and less time the more that you use it. Imagine a solution that transforms your brain's ability to respond to stress with increasing effectiveness and resiliency. Although you may be thinking that such a solution is too good to be true, we assure you that it does exist.

As we're sure you have guessed, the solution we are talking about is the NuCalm technology. Please keep reading to learn how and why it is such an easy and elegant solution to stress, capable of enhancing your life on all levels.

Chapter 3

The NuCalm Story

A Journey of Discovery, Integration and Healing

The NuCalm technology is a revolutionary and synergistic combination of three cutting-edge therapies, each providing its own wide range of health benefits. A fourth component, light blocking, prevents visual stimuli and helps maintain relaxation during treatment.

We will explore each of these components in detail in the next chapter. Here, we want to introduce you to the man who invented NuCalm. His name is Dr. G. Blake Holloway. In the following interview, he shares how and why he created this technology.

Dr. Holloway is a neuroscientist and clinical naturopath, with education in functional biology, clinical nutrition, orthomolecular medicine, applied psychobiology, behavioral science, biophysics (including electro and magnetic therapies), addictionology and acupuncture.

"I was the kid who asked the questions that seemed to trouble people," he said. "I had a little bit of a reputation for annoying teachers because I didn't always accept simple explanations. For example, if I wanted to know why something operated the way it did and was told 'That's because that's the way it is,' I would persist by asking 'Well, why don't we know more?' In many respects, I've always had an insatiable curiosity. I think I'm very internal and I'm extremely visual. I would draw machines as a kid. I wasn't exactly Leonardo da Vinci, but I always wanted to know how something worked."

It was this curiosity, coupled with a keen desire to help others, that led Dr. Holloway to develop the NuCalm technology, adapting it over time. "The impetus that led to its creation was one of need," he said. "I was looking for a solution to a problem. I wasn't seeking to create something with the idea of creating a company. That was far, far from my mind."

Throughout his career, two primary interests have guided Dr. Holloway's work: traumatic stress responses and addictive diseases. "These interests go all the way to my childhood," he said. "On my father's side of the family I watched both of my uncles actually die from alcohol poisoning. My father supported not only our family, but my uncles' families as well.

"My uncles suffered from the most addictive type of alcoholism you can have, which even among alcoholics is relatively rare. It's characterized by intense cravings, as in the example of a person who puts the bottle to his lips and does not take it away until it's empty. That's how it was with my uncles, and I saw the pain my cousins suffered as a result of that. I became very interested in what causes alcoholism and other addictions, and wanted to find out all that could be done to treat people who suffered with addictive disease."

Because of this interest, Dr. Holloway gravitated toward working in addiction treatment centers, rising to upper management positions at a number of centers considered the most sophisticated in their treatment approaches. "The problem, however, was that these centers were not really taking a neuroscientific approach to what they were doing," he said. At that time, the typical standard of care was based on 12-step programs, he said, coupled perhaps with cognitive behavioral therapy.

As Dr. Holloway became aware of neuroscience research related to addiction, stress and anxiety, he wanted to incorporate practical applications of those findings into the centers where he worked. "I got more than a little bit of pushback on that," he said. "In some of the better treatment centers, they would have the doctors give the patients lectures with some information about the brain-related aspects of addiction, but even today there is not a single place that I can point where their treatment modality for addiction is brain-based."

Dr. Holloway said he was determined to find a better way, adding, "One of the things you find in the field of addiction treatment, particularly if you work in it for a long time, is the extremely high rate of relapse. By its very nature and the way that it operates bio-logically, addiction is a relapsing disease. I became interested in in-vestigating the dynamics of that, and developed a clinical reputation for being the go-to guy for relapse. There is just no way that a person will not have relapse from an addictive disease if the fixations in their brain and nervous system are not addressed, but it is so painful and expensive.

"Those fixed set points in the brain and nervous system are what continue to drive the addict's anxiety, worry and depression. They also limit problem-solving ability. If you can get people's nervous systems operating better and offer them a way to be out of that anxiety, then they have a much better chance of being able to heal their addiction and minimize their risk of relapse. I began to search for ways to do that."

In 1998, Dr. Holloway found a clue in his search for a better solution to treat addiction. A PBS television special called "The Hijacked Brain," part of series by noted journalist Bill Moyers entitled *Addiction: Close To Home*, focused on the neuroscience related to addiction. It featured profiles of scientists who were, according to the program's liner notes, "charting the physiological changes that take place in the brain as drugs kick in."

Those who work with addicts are all too aware of these changes, according to Dr. Holloway. "If you look at a more chronically relapsing group," he said, "and if you divide out what the triggering issues are in that group, you find that the primary drivers for relapse are stress and anxiety.

"If you happen to be a person with an addictive disease, and you also have a co-morbid anxiety, you're walking on a real tightrope wire. One of the things used to treat anxiety disorders is a class of drugs known as benzodiazepines. These drugs, by themselves, can have quite an addictive potential, particular-ly among people whose anxiety disorder is very acute. Knowing all of this, as I began my initial investigations, I asked myself what could be brought to the table to better serve these patients."

Treating Medical Conditions and Addiction

Dr. Holloway was concerned, as well, with the discrepancy in how the medical community typically viewed addiction.

"Everyone agrees these days that, when we talk about addiction, we are talking about a medical condition," he said. "However, if you have, for example, congestive heart failure that causes you to be hospitalized a number of times, the medical staff at the hospital would not say 'You've relapsed multiple times with this congestive heart failure, and we just can't continue to deal with you if you keep doing that.' Nevertheless, that is typically how people with addictions are treated. In fact, if addicts are agitated enough during their treatment, they often are summarily discharged from the treatment center, which is a little bit like being discharged from a coronary care center because you had another heart attack.

"I found this outrageous. People would call addiction a disease, yet addiction patients would not get the same respect for their disease problems that they would if they had any other diagnosis in another disease category."

Frustrated by this dynamic, Dr. Holloway spoke out against it. "I got crosswise with some of the institutions I was working at," he said, "because I was trying to push the edge and bring in treatment processes and techniques that could prove more effective. What we were doing at the time, for the most part, was not working.

"For example, take someone in an addiction rehabilitation center. Depending on their condition when they are first admitted, they might spend four days in a detox bed. Then, all of a sudden one day, they find themselves sitting in a chair in a circle for group therapy. Most people under such circumstances find that their thinking and brain processes are a long, long way from being able to be in that kind of learning dynamic. Other than a brief, medically supervised detoxification program, patients weren't really getting the information they needed in what I call the hardware part of the problem.

"If your brain has been subjected to the chemicals and toxins of addictive substances, even though you may be detoxified, you're not cognitively in shape to accomplish very much on your fourth or fifth day in a treatment setting, which primarily consists of lectures and group therapies. I thought it was absolutely outrageous not to be doing more of what I call brain-based modalities.

"One of the things you learn very quickly if you study stress dynamics is: the higher the stress, the poorer the blood flow is to the prefrontal and frontal parts of the brain. These areas are where you can make the most intelligent decisions and where learning takes place. For alcohol and drug treatment to be truly effective, this has to be taken into account. However, it takes time, often more time than is allowed during a typical rehab stint.

"We have a very strange set of circumstances where third party insurance payers got into a mode of approving 28 days of treatment. That number was pulled more or less out of the air. It was based on what they could get insurance companies to pay, not necessarily on how well the patient was progressing. Unfortunately, for-profit people got into the addiction treatment industry early on. There was a lot of money to be made. Then managed care came along and they managed to pay as little as they could on a daily rate. Treatment providers were bidding against each other for the best rate to the insurance companies. When economics dominate treatment modalities, the patients suffer the consequences."

As economic pressures reduced treatment time and quality, Dr. Holloway became even more concerned about patients going into relapse.

"Treatment centers were having a great deal of relapse problems. Their approaches were very formulaic," he said. "I could see that little was being done to address the patients' stress and anxiety, particularly anticipatory anxiety. Many people come into treatment with their social relations frayed, with their employment relations frayed, and very often with legal problems such as drug possession and DWIs. They have a tremendous amount of stress about that.

"If you start looking at people with addictive diseases, you'll notice that they are wired a lot tighter than other people. I began to look for strategies that would address this anxiety in a safer way, because you have so many traumatized patients.

"Plus, there is a period of about a year when people are recovering and the brain is healing, where they may experience what is known as post-acute withdrawal episodes. For a day or two, they might be very vulnerable because the brain is still in the process of sorting itself out.

"Additionally, in people with addictive disease, there is a biological component that can be passed on. You can have what we call adult children of alcoholics who will end up with problems of their own. The kinds of chaotic families they grew up in presented a real challenge to achieving their developmental milestones. These children experience a lot of stress and anxiety. Because of that, their problem-solving ability can be greatly diminished."

Steps Along the Way

In his quest to find more effective addiction treatments, Dr. Holloway explored brain wave biofeedback, also known as neurofeedback or neurotherapy.

After studies[1] conducted in the 1960s and 1970s, Drs. Gene Peniston and Paul Kulkosky developed alpha-theta brain wave biofeedback, using peripheral temperature training protocols and computerized electroencephalograph biofeedback equipment. It helps normalize brain wave states and increase alpha and theta brain waves, both of which are associated with optimal mental function and increased levels of pleasure, insight and creativity.

Research has demonstrated[2] that individuals prone to addiction often do not produce enough alpha-theta brain waves, predisposing them to addictive substances that artificially and temporarily produce feelings of relaxation.

Patients who underwent brain wave biofeedback therapy showed better brain wave management and naturally produced more alpha-theta waves. Over time, this improved their decision-making abilities and enabled them to experience contentment and well-being more regularly. Thus, brain wave therapy was an effective tool for treating addiction and preventing relapse, as well for treating depression, anxiety and other mental health conditions.

"Brain wave biofeedback had really great promise," Dr. Holloway said, "so I underwent a lot of advanced training in it. In the 1980s, Dr. Peniston and Dr. Kulkosky conducted interesting research within the Veterans Administration, including taking a group of alcoholic Vietnam-era veterans, who also had PTSD, through a series of brain wave biofeedback sessions.[3] This small group of people really cleared up, and had some stunning results with resolving the PTSD. The problem they had, however, was that it took anywhere from 45 to 65 treatments to achieve those results. Even though they were successful in this one VA hospital in Texas, none of the other VA hospitals and institutions picked it up and used it."

As Dr. Holloway began to use brain wave biofeedback therapy on patients, he found that it produced positive benefits for anxiety. "We were seeing some extraordinary results with brain wave biofeedback," he said, "including help for traumatic brain injuries. As a matter of fact, a Texas legislator's daughter who had been in a car wreck was treated with brain wave biofeedback. Her father got it written into law that insurance companies had to pay for brain wave biofeedback therapy for traumatic brain injuries in Texas."

One of the principles of brain wave biofeedback therapy, according to Dr. Holloway, is its operant conditioning. "It's Pavlovian. What you're essentially doing with brain wave biofeedback, when you hit the target brain wave, is getting a reward," he said. "You can set up the parameters that you want, and the reward occurs when the outcome you are seeking is attained. Our brains have a great capacity for learning, but not if they are stuck in a certain way. Brain wave biofeedback helps to clear up the brain. As I began to work with it, I could see the clinical stabilizations that it was achieving with my patients.

"But much of what I learned was more about what is going on within the brain, particularly at the cellular level. With brain wave biofeedback, you use sensors on the scalp that are reading the electricity underneath the scalp, on the surface of the brain. The technology is sophisticated enough that you could measure the brain wave patterns in a baby's brain. If the child's parents were alcoholics, you could actually pick up an aberration in the baby's brain waves in what is called the P300 range. I had some interesting successes with brain wave biofeedback therapy, but it was extremely time consuming and it was expensive for the patient."

Around this same time, research underway in London and at the Menninger Clinic in Topeka, Kansas, drew the attention of Dr. Holloway.

"These researchers were doing some very interesting stuff. They were examining advanced meditators and yogis from India who had such control over their nervous system that they could change their heart rate at will," he said. "They could take their breath rate down to about a breath a minute. It takes a tremendous amount of training and discipline to accomplish that.

"The Menninger Clinic was beginning to look at the EEGs of the brains[4] of these people. You could see what I would call extraordinary states of consciousness. That research has evolved into what is called contemplative neuroscience, which is an actual branch of neuroscience today.

"Incidentally, what NuCalm does within a few daily sessions is what patients treated within a contemplative neuroscience framework take an average of 90 days to achieve, meaning positive plastic changes within the brain, which is known as *neuroplasticity*.

"One of the other interests I picked up while I was looking at these different biofeedback techniques was something called respiratory sinus arrhythmia training. Today it is called heart rate variability. I trained with a number of pioneers in HRV biofeedback, which is driven by breath and focus control. As we worked with it, we learned that you could shift people's autonomic nervous systems to the better side of the equation.

"When you start looking at anxiety and stress, you must look at the autonomic nervous system. There are two sides to the autonomic nervous system, the sympathetic and the parasympathetic. The sympathetic is related to what is known as fight-or-flight, and the parasympathetic is related to what we call rest-and-restore or

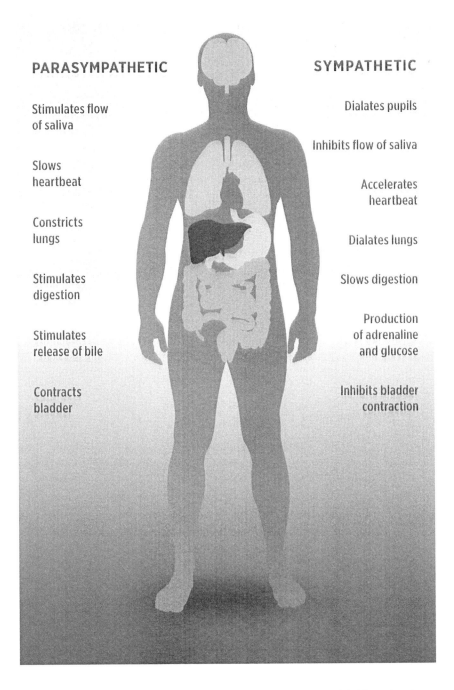

PARASYMPATHETIC

Stimulates flow
of saliva

Slows
heartbeat

Constricts
lungs

Stimulates
digestion

Stimulates
release of bile

Contracts
bladder

SYMPATHETIC

Dialates pupils

Inhibits flow of saliva

Accelerates
heartbeat

Dialates lungs

Slows digestion

Production
of adrenaline
and glucose

Inhibits bladder
contraction

How the Autonomic Nervous System Interacts with Your Body

rest-and-digest. As I worked with addicts and kept records, I found that patients who could stabilize their HRV into a positive zone, a zone that we call coherent, did not have problems and we could eliminate them from the relapse group if they kept up the practice."

Next to pique Dr. Holloway's interest was the work of Dr. Margaret Patterson of Great Britain. She had a following among rock stars and heavy metal bands of the day, including Eric Clapton and Pete Townshend, both of whom she treated for substance abuse problems. In 1969, after having learned how electro-acupuncture treatments significantly reduced withdrawal symptoms of opiate addiction, Dr. Patterson developed a form of *cranial electrotherapy stimulation*, known as CES, which she called NeuroElectric Therapy. A non-acupuncture, non-pharmacological intervention for addiction treatment, NET was delivered via a device dubbed the black box, due to its appearance. NET controlled and modulated CES output waveforms, allowing patients to detoxify rapidly and effectively from addictive substances including heroin, cocaine, methadone, nicotine and alcohol.

Intrigued by her work, Dr. Holloway decided to investigate CES in general.

"I had an opportunity to spend some time in St. Petersburg, in the Soviet Union. That is where CES was invented," he said. "I went to a week-long conference where researchers were presenting their findings. At that time, there was even a lot of work with electro-anesthesia because conventional anesthesia was very expensive in the Soviet Union. I was able to meet a couple of scientists who had been involved in producing different CES devices. These devices were introduced into the U.S. and had a brief popularity in a few addiction therapy facilities. Some patients achieved great results using them, but overall the result level was very unpredictable. Yet I could see there was something important happening."

Not only did Dr. Holloway want to know more about CES and addiction treatment, he sought more information about its benefits for treating trauma and chronic pain. "That's another area of addiction that's absolutely tragic," he said. "If you've got chronic pain and you go into an addiction treatment center, if you ask for something to relieve that pain, even for a headache, you'll be told that you're drug seeking. It's quite inexcusable."

Dr. Holloway acquired every kind of CES device that was available at the time. "I even built a few myself," he said, "and it was clear that something was happening, but also that something was still missing."

Seeking more answers, Dr. Holloway had what he described as a "lucky stumble" when he became aware of *neurotransmitter* lab testing.

"When we finally achieved the ability to test neurotransmitters… that was one of the breakthroughs that started bringing everything together for me," he said. "You can't test neurotransmitters in the brain; you can only look at them systemically. Then in the 1990s, testing evolved that allowed you to measure neurotransmitter metabolites, or waste products, and develop algorithms to be able to study the metabolites of neurotransmitters. This, in turn, provides us with a way to determine a body-based range for the neurotransmitters.

"One of the things we started to see quite clearly as neurotransmitter science evolved was that neurotransmitter status had a great deal to do with addictive diseases. People who are very low in serotonin, for example, will have a higher level of craving. If two people crave a beer and one of them is an alcoholic, one of them can have one beer and feel satisfied, but the alcoholic has very low serotonin and may require six beers to have something even near the same satisfaction level.

"As I began to look at this from a holistic approach, I began to investigate amino acid supplementation because every neurotransmitter in the brain has a composite amino acid that is the raw material from which the neurotransmitter is formed. Tryptophan is used by the body to produce serotonin, tyrosine is used to produce dopamine, and so forth.

"Dopamine is hyper-released from the ventral tegmental area of the brain, and it drives craving, addiction and euphoric recall. When dopamine is released in the addictive process, you have a psychological euphoric recall. In addiction, it's often said that people want to feel as good as the first time they heavily drank, and that is a part of euphoric recall. It's the feel-good sensation that comes from the hyper-release of dopamine. The pleasure one gets from alcohol or a drug is driven by a very hyper dopamine release from this area of the brain, and that is true of all people who end up with addiction.

"Stress, as it turns out, particularly if you had a stressful childhood, is one of the causes that creates hypersensitivity in the ventral tegmental area. Furthermore, at the circuit level of the brain, what's going on in these chronic stress levels is the same thing that's going on when the thermostat in your home is broken. If you set your home thermostat for 74 degrees, once that level is reached, a signal should go back to the furnace or air conditioner indicating that the target goal has been reached, which tells the unit to shut off. That's what we call a negative feedback loop. When the thermostat is broken, this doesn't occur.

"In the brain, the negative feedback loop runs from the hypo-thalamus to the anterior pituitary gland, which then sends a signal to the adrenal glands to release a large category of stimulatory chemicals such as norepinephrine, which we know as adrenaline, during times of stress. That doesn't shut off in people with high anxiety because they don't have an effective negative feedback loop.

"The system we have in our brain to help things not get overheated and overexcited is the GABA system. GABA is inhibitory and is essential to autonomic nervous system balance, what we would call stress management. Serotonin is also inhibitory in the brain. Once we were able to measure neurotransmitters, I worked with a large base of research subjects who had multiple relapse issues.

"One of the early things I found, which was pretty startling to me as I looked at this trying to fit all the pieces of the puzzle together, was that there were two highly opposite conditions in people with high anxiety. In some people, I would find a linear relationship with low amounts of GABA, and then in other people who were also highly anxious, I would find extremely high amounts of GABA.

"Now why is someone with high amounts of GABA anxious? They should be very calm. Well, the reason is that the GABA is not actually reaching the receptor sites where it needs to act. I had a lab that was assisting me with this, and it became very clear that people with anxiety had different problems.

"Continuing my research, I took some of these people with really high GABA numbers and did CES treatments with them. When the specimens came back, all of a sudden those high numbers were gone. Well, where did all that GABA go? We believe it went into the receptor sites because one of the things that CES does is help make membranes in the cells of the brain a little bit more permeable so that it is easier for substances to pass through the membrane into the cell. This is what is necessary for the neurotransmitters to attach to the correct binding site.

"Then I thought to myself, if benzodiazepines actually work to upregulate the activity of GABA, how can we get the brain to do that on its own? So I began to put together some formulas and, after about a year, we were really getting some significant clinical results. We could monitor and map the anxiety levels and crisis levels in people, and we found what we were doing was making a big difference. It was clear that certain people were really responding to CES treatments, but CES can't create the neurotransmitters. If you combine the amino acids with the CES, it absolutely jump-starts the system."

As Dr. Holloway's research and discoveries progressed, he entered into a relationship with one of the dentists responsible for introducing conscious sedation to the dental field, where some highly fearful patients had to be tranquilized with intravenous drugs before treatment was possible.

"I really didn't know anything about dentistry," Dr. Holloway said, "but that is how we got connected to the dental anxiety problem. Statistics still show that around 60 million people don't go to the dentist because of high anxiety. Many of those people have what I call medical PTSD from their childhood experiences with dentists.

"We worked with over 13,000 people in an initial clinical investigation project. By combining CES with amino acid therapy, we were able to handle a large number of these patients without intravenous sedation. And if we combined what we were doing with nitrous oxide, it was equivalent to any kind of IV sedation."

Due to the advancements in brain wave biofeedback equipment, Dr. Holloway could record brain mappings of dental patients involved in this project, which he used for further research. He began studying *evoked potentials*, the brain's responses to specific stimuli.

"When doing brain wave biofeedback to help with stress, anxiety, trauma and addiction, you want to get what are known as *alpha-theta crossovers*. The evoked potential that I was working with was audio-visual," he said. "For example, I would flash light in someone's eyes at 10 cycles a second, which is what an alpha wave does, and after a short while that person's brain would go into 10 cycles per second.

"You can also do auditory evocation, so I began to experiment with *binaural beats*, which operate on what is called *frequency-following response* and which have been scientifically proven to evoke potential.

"One day I decided to do all of these together. What was very interesting was that if I did alpha-theta frequencies auditorily, combined with the amino acids and the CES, I began to see that many episodes of alpha-theta frequencies were taking place. What we found was that, very rapidly, usually within the first or second session, patients were achieving results that would take 20 episodes of brain wave biofeedback alone. All of the subjects were showing great improvement, including some agoraphobics and people with really acute anxiety responses.

"Then, when we started measuring the subjects' heart rate variability, we found that we could very quickly stabilize them into a parasympathetic response, which is most conducive to overall health."

Light blocking is NuCalm's final component. Dr. Holloway had learned during his work with brain wave biofeedback that, when we close our eyes, the brain begins to generate alpha waves automatically.

"The occipital part of your brain at the back of your head is where your vision happens," he said. "You don't see with your eyes. Your eyes only collect light. It's your brain that makes the picture.

"You can use an EEG and have people close their eyes. If you have sensors on the occipital region, you'll see the alpha waves go up. It's almost like a free gift we can give ourselves to help ourselves relax. That's one of the reasons why you see meditators with their eyes closed.

"I found I could get up to a 30 percent increase in alpha waves simply by having people close their eyes and then block light with an eye mask. In rooms where dental surgeries occur, as well as in many other types of operating rooms, there is usually very bright light, which can make it difficult to relax. I would try to get the patients to use black out masks because it would make them much more relaxed."

NuCalm Is Born

Dr. Holloway's journey to develop the NuCalm technology spanned 12 years of slow, steady progress. He kept experimenting and augmenting what he was doing with new discoveries, as he continued trying to help people along the way. As new scientific developments occurred in related research, he would investigate, test and validate their usefulness and effectiveness then, where appropriate, add them to the system. Throughout this time, he continued to work with a variety of patients.

"When I originally started this, I was seeking a solution for people with addictive diseases who also suffered from co-morbid anxiety disorders," he said. The work led him to sufferers of PTSD and other types of trauma, as well as the dental patients mentioned before.

Dr. Holloway found all different types of patients affected by high degrees of stress and anxiety. He recounted how, early on, a simple biofeedback technique played a role in his search.

"I remember being in a treatment center and sharing this technique with patients. It's a very basic technique," he said. "What you do is place a thermometer between your thumb and forefinger. You can use any sort of inexpensive thermometer that you can buy at any drug store. As you hold it, you relax and imagine that your hand is warming up. If you are successful, as the temperature of your hand goes up, your vascular peripheral circulation will become better. That can't happen, of course, unless you can put yourself into a parasympathetic state. When you're in a sympathetic state, your peripheral circulation is very poor."

As this chapter has discussed, people suffering from high degrees of stress and anxiety are typically unable to put themselves into a parasympathetic state. Helping them to do so was one of Dr. Holloway's goals, beginning with his research in brain wave biofeedback therapy.

"What I finally arrived at is the ability to create within the brain those preferential frequencies and doing it in an evoked way, rather than just in an operant conditioning way," Dr. Holloway said. "This occurred most effectively when we combined the auditory part (the neuroacoustic software) that is a form of evoked potential, with the CES, the amino acid formula, and a light-blocking mask or dark glasses. They all work in concert with each other to highly potentiate the autonomic system toward the parasympathetic state."

About halfway through what he calls his clinical proving stage, Dr. Holloway had compiled patient feedback on his treatments and realized he was on the verge of developing a new, proprietary system for successfully dealing with the health issues he originally had hoped to resolve.

"Looking back, I think it was after I'd worked with about 50 patients in a dental setting that I knew we had something very powerful," he said. "It still needed refinements. At that time, I hadn't finished developing the final amino acid formula, but I knew I had figured out a solution to stress and anxiety."

By this time, much of Dr. Holloway's focus was on upregulating the GABA system in as powerful a way as possible. "I remember a very seminal day when I got really excited," he said. "We were looking at lab results, EEGs and heart rate variability. We had six people to sample that day and three of them demonstrated between a 100 to 200 percent increase in HRV, which is a portal into the health of the human autonomic nervous system. So I knew we had found a sweet spot if we could continue to produce these types of results."

Dr. Holloway then realized the system he was developing had much greater potential than he initially had considered. "That's when I started thinking a lot bigger," he said. "Once I saw how the system I had developed could balance the autonomic nervous system, I became confident that it could be effective for treating a wide range of diseases related to autonomic dysfunction."

Autonomic nervous system dysfunction, or *dysautonomia,*

negatively affects the nerves that carry information from the brain and spinal cord to the heart, bladder, intestines, sweat glands, pupils, blood vessels and especially the vagus nerve.

There is a wide range of health concerns created by autonomic dysfunction, which might include excessive fatigue and thirst, excessively high or low blood pressure, irregular heart rates, difficulties breathing or swallowing, constipation and other gastrointestinal problems, bladder and urinary problems, and sexual problems such as erectile dysfunction in men or vaginal dryness and orgasm difficulties in women. Autonomic dysfunction also can be a factor in chronic fatigue syndrome, fibromyalgia, irritable bowel syndrome and interstitial cystitis.

The area of the brain that regulates all of these functions contains a group of motor neurons known as the *nucleus ambiguus,* which Dr. Holloway described as "the Nile source point of the entire vagus nerve system." Because of Dr. Holloway's research, we now know that NuCalm has a highly positive effect on this brain region.

Just as important to Dr. Holloway as the test results, however, were the overwhelmingly positive responses from patients as he introduced them to the NuCalm technology.

"I remember one man in particular," he said. "He was a pretty wealthy guy, and had been to treatment over a dozen consecutive times for his alcohol problem. He was really struggling, and you could see that by how out of balance his initial HRV test was.

"Once we completed his first NuCalm session, he looked at me and said, 'I don't know how to explain this, but something has changed in me big time.' He worked with me for about three months and did not relapse at any time during that period. In point of fact, he had a surprising trauma resolution with a past issue in his life that he had never shared with me. That just sticks out as one of those high points because this guy was just really, really distressed. Because of NuCalm, something shifted and moved him off of his craving and his euphoric recall.

"This man was a very Type A person and it was amazing to watch him go through that transition. He really took to NuCalm and became a part of a group that used to come to my outpatient addiction sessions. I had a moral support group, and all of these folks would come for our version of happy hour. They would come between 4:30 and 5:30 p.m. and sit in lounge chairs, then we would use NuCalm for an hour before the group discussion. What I noticed were two things: the group discussions were very relaxed and insightful, and we rarely had an empty chair. So we integrated that into our addiction program.

"I didn't realize it at the time, but what we were doing was really contemplative neuroscience. That was a long time before the term was even used because it wasn't yet recognized. But today it's an exciting branch of the overall field of neuroscience, with ongoing research being conducted at universities such as the University of California at San Francisco, the University of Wisconsin and Harvard."

This is another example of Dr. Holloway being ahead of his time.

Near the end of his 12-year NuCalm development journey, Dr. Holloway began considering whether the system could be of service to the public for personal use, beyond his clinical treatment.

"From the start, I was simply looking to improve clinical outcomes," he said. "I began my journey looking for solutions to improve treatment for addictive disease with an emphasis on stress management, but the outcome ended up being an all-natural solution for maintaining and balancing the health of the human autonomic nervous system.

"Sometimes people decide they want to invent something and then they set about doing so. With NuCalm, it was not like that. It really was an evolution and it was quite late in the game that I realized that we might be able to do something beyond my clinical practice. Everything was being driven forward by the discoveries that were being made at the time, both through my concerted efforts and those of others, but they weren't being drawn to the same place.

"Upon reflection, I was putting together a puzzle that previously wasn't being worked on by anyone. Maybe it was my holistic approach, maybe it was my continued curiosity to explore new ideas, or maybe it was simply a determination to succeed out of compassion for the people I was determined to help.

"What we have assembled in NuCalm are things from really different boxes, as it were. One of things about me is I tend to climb up on the ladder and look over the edge of one box into other boxes and think to myself, 'What would be fun and interesting to take from those other boxes and experiment with?'

"That's what I did as I came to develop NuCalm. I drew from these different boxes, or areas of research, that weren't considered to be related at the time, and I integrated them to create something new. What we ended up with was something that could create a predictable, fast acting, safe and positive clinical response.

"Recently, I began investigating the latest research in physics and neuroscience and have created a totally new neuroacoustic method of auditory brain entrainment, based on that research. It's nonlinear and dynamical, which is physics terminology. What it means is that the auditory tone oscillates or vibrates, instead of being syncopated like binaural beats. This is a much more complex and sophisticated method for producing brain entrainment and will be a part of NuCalm 2.0, with patent pending. Initially, four new music tracks will be released using this proprietary software. Whichever NuCalm version you use, though, you will achieve relaxation."

"The NuCalm technology is the negative feedback loop that you need to shift the autonomic nervous system into a state of balance, with improved parasympathetic functioning.

"In that sense, it's really bio-mimetic, meaning we've made a biological mimic of something that's absolutely naturalistic in the body. Rather than it being something external and non-native to the human physiology, everything we have in NuCalm is somewhat native. We're not using outside drugs to do this. We're providing the body and mind with the necessary building blocks and raw materials to create the positive results that we want. The body and mind know how to relax. We are simply facilitating the process, and making it easy and predictable."

Summing up his feelings about the efficiency and transformative power of the system he created, Dr. Holloway said, "What I think is probably the greatest attribute of this invention is that, without my having to sit down with you to undergo a lot of training and a lot of coaching, you can use it to significantly improve your brain and your autonomic nervous system functioning…beginning immediately, with your first few sessions using the system on your own.

"I've spent a lot of time in monasteries and other places for meditation. I've met people who are really committed to their meditation practices, yet neither they nor their instructors hope to have a lot happen for at least three to five years.

"Well, guess what? With NuCalm, looking at the EEG, we can see people's brains go, within minutes, where advanced meditators spend years training their brains to go.

"What we are creating, by providing this mimic of the negative feedback loop in the brain's hypothalamic-pituitary-adrenal axis, is the ability for NuCalm users to reach that same level of detachment and create the same brain wave patterns as advanced meditators.

"They've been doing advanced medical meditation studies since the 1970s and researchers continue to do this research today, both in the mental health field and in the area of contemplative neuroscience. Researchers are taking individuals with long-term mental health issues that have not been too responsive to other treatments and, after 90 days of what is essentially meditation and contemplative work, they're finding positive plastic changes in the subjects' brains.

"With NuCalm, you can achieve those same benefits much more quickly," Dr. Holloway concluded. "Your brain can enter into the same state as an advanced Zen meditator, in just one or two sessions with NuCalm and with limited effort. This technology is a tool for shifting you into those optimal brain and relaxation states, and when that shift happens, you really do see transformation."

Chapter 4

How and Why NuCalm Works

In this chapter, we are going to explain why NuCalm is so effective for predictably achieving two vitally important health benefits, stress relief and restorative sleep.

"With NuCalm, we have a singular purpose: to improve quality of life by lowering stress and improving sleep quality without drugs," said Jim Poole, CEO of Solace Lifesciences, the company that produces this technology. "Unfortunately, between our food sources barely being food anymore, and the stress and the pace of our culture around the globe, we are not getting the restorative sleep we need, which is accelerating each and every disease state that we know of, especially autoimmune diseases."

As you learned in Chapter 2, stress refers to any physical, chemical or emotional factor causing physical or mental tension that can disrupt the body's equilibrium, thus acting as a primary trigger in the disease process. Stress results in anxiety and inflammation, which are all part of the human condition. Yet they are known to cause chemical and structural changes in every system of the body, including the circulatory, digestive, endocrine and nervous systems.

Each of us copes with it differently, but stress is universally damaging to cells and is a precursor and catalyst to numerous diseases. To maintain health, you must eat a healthy diet, perform regular exercise, effectively manage stress and achieve autonomic nervous system balance through restorative sleep.

NuCalm is the first and only therapeutic method in the world to receive a U.S. patent "for balancing and maintaining the health of the human autonomic nervous system."

Through biochemical and electrical signaling, NuCalm mimics the body's own processes for preparing to relax deeply, naturally bringing brain waves to the pre-sleep state of consciousness, which are the alpha and theta stages of sleep. For this reason, NuCalm has been likened to "meditation in a box."

Typically, within a few minutes, NuCalm achieves this deeply relaxed, meditative state by shifting the body into sustained parasympathetic nervous system dominance. This is the only time your body is capable of deep regeneration and repair.

By using the NuCalm technology, you enable your body to restore its cellular health, resolve neuromuscular tension, increase mental acuity, enhance sleep stability, increase energy levels, improve stress resiliency, regulate circadian rhythm, and improve overall health and wellness.

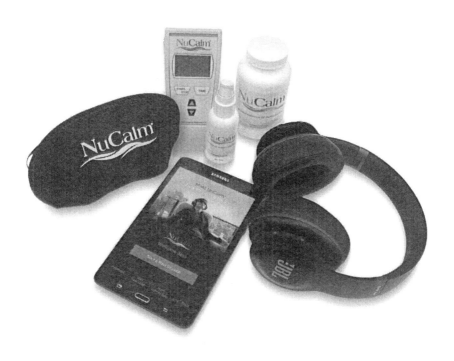

The Four Components of NuCalm

To fully grasp how and why NuCalm provides these benefits, we need to further explore each of the four components researched and integrated into the system by Dr. Holloway.

As you learned in Chapter 3, NuCalm's four components are its proprietary neuroacoustic software, cranial electrotherapy stimulation, a proprietary amino acid nutritional formula available as a supplement or cream, and a means for light blocking. What follows is an overview of how each of these elements works with the body.

Component One: Neuroacoustics and Binaural Beats

Though the terms *neuroacoustics* and binaural beats may be unfamiliar to you, research in this field dates back to the early 19th century. Simply put, neuroacoustics make use of binaural beats to initiate changes in brain wave patterns, many having significant therapeutic value. Binaural beats involve different neurological pathways than those normally used for hearing. Typically, the beats are delivered using headphones, with one sound frequency played in the left ear and a different frequency played in the right ear.

German scientist Heinrich Wilhelm Dove first discovered binaural beats and their effects, and in 1839 published a paper about his research in the scientific journal *Repertorium der Physik*.[1] The scientific community, however, largely ignored his work.

That changed in 1973, when Gerald Oster published an article in *Scientific American* entitled "Auditory Beats in the Brain," which identified and compiled the various old and new research projects on binaural beats that had occurred in the century following Dove's findings. Oster included his own insights into the potential of binaural beats for research in the cognitive and neurological fields, and as a tool for medical diagnosis and therapy.[2]

Following the publication of Oster's paper, broadcaster Robert Monroe, physicist Thomas Campbell and electrical engineer Dennis

Mennerich began researching binaural beats for potential effects on both conscious and altered brain states, including out-of-body experiences. Monroe and his colleagues soon discovered that binaural beats did facilitate altered states of consciousness and corresponding shifts in brain wave patterns.

As part of this research,[3] Monroe conducted thousands of experiments using an EEG machine to monitor his test subjects' electrical brain wave patterns. These experiments showed that binaural beats could influence brain wave frequencies. Additionally, Monroe found that the brain did not respond just in the area of hearing, or in one hemisphere or the other. Rather, the entire brain resonated. The brain waves in both brain hemispheres exhibited identical frequencies, amplitude and coherence. To further this work, he established the Monroe Institute, a nonprofit binaural beat research and education center. Monroe was largely responsible for creating the personal development industry of binaural beats and neuroacoustics.

The effects of binaural beats are produced mainly in an area of the brain known as the *superior olivary nucleus*. Both the right and left superior olivary nuclei play primary roles in multiple hearing processes and are important to the pathways of our body's auditory system. Binaural (which means both ears) beats result from the interaction between auditory tones of different frequencies being played in each ear. Research[4] shows that to be effective, the tones must register below 1,000 *hertz*, or cycles per second, and differ in frequency between 1 to 30 Hz.

What effects these beats have on brain waves depend on the difference in frequencies between the two tones. For example, if a pure tone of 300 Hz is presented to the right ear and a pure tone of 305 Hz is presented simultaneously to the left ear, an amplitude-modulated standing wave of 5 Hz is experienced within the superior olivary nuclei, as the two tones mesh in and out of phase.

This 5 Hz wave is undetected as sound by the listener because humans can only hear in the range of 20 to 20,000 Hz. Instead, it is perceived by the brain as an auditory beat. These beats can be used to entrain specific neural rhythms, thus modulating brain wave frequencies.

Binaural beats affect the brain and the autonomic nervous system by influencing brain functions in ways beyond those related to hearing. This influencing effect is known as both *frequency-following response* and *brain wave entrainment*.

When binaural beats are perceived, they create a stimulus within the overall frequency range of brain waves (high beta, beta, alpha, theta and delta). As the process unfolds, the frequency of the binaural

Human Brain Wave Patterns

Your brain cycles through different brain wave states each day, depending on what you are dealing with, both internally and externally, at any particular moment. Each of these brain wave states has its own pattern, frequency and amplitude that can be measured using EEG monitoring.

What follows is a list of the most common brain wave states, their EEG frequency correlations and their associated psychological and physiological states:

High Beta (23 to 38 Hz) — fear and anxiety

Beta (13 to 30 Hz) — day-to-day wakefulness

Alpha (8 to 12 Hz) — relaxation, meditation, idleness

Theta (4 to 7 Hz) — sleep, healing, lost sense of time and place

Delta (0.5 to 3 Hz) — deep, dreamless sleep.

While you are awake, alpha-theta brain wave states support creativity and learning, and offer the greatest opportunity to relax, restore and heal. Alpha-theta crossover events occur in the state of pre-sleep, where much of NuCalm's benefits happen.

Regular use of the NuCalm system literally trains your brain to shift more easily, predictably and verifiably into deeply healing states of relaxation. This strengthens your body's resiliency and stress-coping mechanisms.

beats causes the brain's own wave patterns to resonate at that same frequency, creating the entrainment effect. In the example above, the brain will start to resonate and entrain to the beat frequency of 5 Hz. That falls within the theta brain wave zone, which is a state of deep, restorative sleep and healing. If the beat frequency changes, the brain responds by following the frequency change.

Many researchers have verified the entrainment effect. Dr. Holloway and Solace Lifesciences, as well as others, have conducted research demonstrating that the frequency-following response activates various sites in the brain, including the prefrontal and frontal cortices.[5,6,7] This can bring about a harmonization between the left and right hemispheres of the brain, sometimes referred to as brain hemisphere synchronization.

Research suggests[8] that use of binaural beats can bring about a re-organization of the brain itself and its neural pathways. This is known as neuroplasticity, which scientists are discovering offers a wide range of healthy cognitive and physiological benefits.

Since the 1970s, research into the various uses and benefits of binaural beats and neuroacoustics has continued to grow. Thus far, the research establishes or suggests that this technology can help enhance attention, relaxation, mood, memory and creativity.[9]

Binaural beats help stimulate the production of various hormones and neurochemicals by entraining brain frequencies to the alpha-theta range. As examples, theta waves are associated with production of cat-echolamine hormones (which include adrenaline, norepinephrine and dopamine) and alpha waves are associated with production of serotonin,[10] a hormone neurotransmitter responsible for balancing mood, among other functions. A deficit of serotonin has been linked to a variety of health conditions including anxiety, depression and sleep problems like insomnia.

The alpha-theta waves induced by binaural beats also have been shown to help treat addiction[11] and anxiety,[12,13] improve learning abilities,[14] and support deep, restful sleep.[15]

Given the above, you can see why neuroacoustics is an essential component of NuCalm. Yet Dr. Holloway did not simply adopt existing neuroacoustic technology. He improved on it for NuCalm, and now has created a new method for NuCalm 2.0, explained in Chapter 3.

The NuCalm proprietary neuroacoustic entrainment software, which uses complex binaural beats and frequency-following response technologies, required significant advances in the design of binaural and monaural beat sound acoustics. It paces brain waves to frequency patterns of alpha and theta, in the 4 to 12 Hz range, which are associated with calm and deep meditation.

NuCalm delivers these alpha-theta frequencies through a stereo headset and within an overlay of soothing classical music. You cannot hear alpha and theta frequencies because the music acts as a carrier wave, but your brain is able to interpret the frequencies' patterns to achieve deep relaxation and rejuvenation. A selection of music tracks either are integrated into the headset or delivered through the NuCalm 2.0 smart device app.

Component Two: Cranial Electrotherapy Stimulation

The use of electricity for healing dates back to ancient times. For example, back in the second century, the famed Greek physician and surgeon Claudius Galen was considered the most accomplished and skillful healer and medical researcher of the Roman Empire. He recommended the use of electrical shocks, through contact with electric eels and other electrogenic fish, as a treatment for a variety of health conditions.

The modern-day medical usage of electrical current dates back to studies conducted in the late 1700s and early 1800s. The researcher Giovanni Aldini, for example, began in 1794 to experiment with low-intensity electrical stimulation in the form of galvanic currents on both animals and humans, including himself. By 1804, Aldini could show that direct low-intensity galvanic currents could successfully treat patients suffering from melancholia (depression).[16]

A century later in 1902, researchers in France conducted the first experiments with low intensity electrical stimulation of the brain. At the time, this treatment was known as electrosleep because of its ability to induce sleep and deep states of restfulness. It was not until the late 1940s and into the 1950s, however, that researchers in the Soviet Union developed what is known now as CES.

This noninvasive therapy involves the application of a low, pulsed electric current at specific sites to stimulate the brain and brainstem. The current itself is very low and normally is not felt by the person receiving CES treatments. In the case of NuCalm, it is 1/10,000th of an amp, which is approximately the same as the cells' own electrical values. Treatments are administered easily, with the current supplied through electrode patches placed on the neck beneath the earlobes.

In the United States, CES is cleared by the Food and Drug Administration to treat anxiety, depression and insomnia. Research also indicates that CES enhances mental focus[17] and suggests benefits in treatment for addiction,[18,19] traumatic brain injury,[20] pain,[21] attention deficit hyperactivity disorder (ADHD),[22] PTSD,[23] Parkinson's Disease[24] and cognition.[25]

Research over the past 60 years indicates that a small amount of the CES current reaches the thalamic region of the brain[26] and facilitates the release of neurotransmitters. Moreover, it improves metabolism of neurotransmitters, as evidenced by an increase in their metabolites.[27]

Other research points to a normalization and balance of the brain's neurochemistry by re-establishing optimal neurotransmitter levels.[28] This occurs as the low-level electrical current interacts with cell membranes, modifying conversion of neurochemicals associated with the brain's classical second messenger pathways. Communication between brain cells and neurons occurs by various complex means, including second messenger pathways and the better-known synapse interactions using neurotransmitters and receptor sites.

Dr. Holloway's research shows that CES opens GABA receptor sites in the brain. This is significant because, as discussed in Chapter 3, the effects of GABA supplementation alone were not always predictable because the receptor sites in some patients were not open. When CES is used in conjunction with GABA supplements, a predictable positive response occurs each time.

Combining both chemical and electrical signaling gives NuCalm its ability to manage both the brain's *amygdala* and the HPA axis, creating the speed and predictability with which its benefits take effect. This is one of the unique features of NuCalm.

Combining CES with precursor neurotransmitters, such as the NuCalm dietary supplements, causes a profound state of relaxation and reduction of anxiety. Quantitative EEGs show a slowing of brain wave activity from beta (high alertness) to alpha-theta (deep meditation) frequencies.

There are no known contraindications to the use of CES, except for persons with a pacemaker, a ventricular assist device or a brain implant. It is safe and convenient to use at home, without professional supervision. It also is safe to use by itself or, as in the case of NuCalm, in tandem with most other health treatments.

Component Three: NuCalm's Proprietary Supplements or Cream

The third component of the NuCalm technology, its proprietary dietary supplement formula, was developed by Dr. Holloway based on his research using amino acid therapy to treat patients suffering from addiction, anxiety, depression and PTSD. Amino acid therapy has been used as a treatment for these and other conditions for decades and, with good reason, continues to grow in popularity.

Amino acids are the basic building blocks your body uses to create neurotransmitters, the biochemical messengers that communicate information throughout your brain and body. Your entire nervous system is regulated almost entirely by amino acids and the neurotransmitters they create. Neurotransmitters are what your brain uses, for example, to send impulses that tell your heart to keep beating and your lungs to breathe. Neurotransmitters also play other important roles in the body because of the ways in which they affect mood, cognitive function, sleep and even your weight.

When neurotransmitters are out of balance or deficient, they can cause or contribute to a wide range of physical and psychological problems, as well as influencing neurological problems such as Parkinson's disease.[29]

Problems such as anxiety, depression, insomnia and pain can originate in the brain due to neurotransmitter imbalances, and amino acid therapy is effective for treating such conditions.[30] However, today's mainstream medical system continues to overlook the value of amino acid therapy.

Many doctors and mental health specialists prescribe drugs such as SSRIs or selective serotonin reuptake inhibitors, SNRIs or selective norepinephrine inhibitors, and benzodiazepines to treat conditions caused or exacerbated by imbalances of amino acids and neurotransmitters. These classes of drugs work by targeting neurotransmitter receptor sites. Ironically, although these drugs can help manage symptoms, they also can negatively affect the body's own ability to produce and properly utilize neurotransmitters.

As the saying goes, no health condition is caused by a drug deficiency. All too often, however, health conditions are caused by amino acid deficiencies or excesses, and their consequent neurotransmitter imbalances. Therefore, it is safer and more effective to address such conditions by restoring amino acid and neurotransmitter balance, which is what amino acid therapy does.

The primary ingredients in NuCalm's dietary formula are a proprietary blend of GABA and L-theanine. GABA is an inhibitory neurotransmitter that reduces the excitability of neurons and promotes a natural state of calm and deep relaxation. Overstimulated or over-active neurons may lead to restlessness, irritability and sleeplessness. GABA inhibits nerve cells from over-firing, thus allowing feelings of calmness and stability.

The body produces GABA from the amino acid glutamine and the sugar glucose. It is concentrated in the midbrain region and plays a role in healthy pituitary function, which helps maintain hormone synthesis, proper sleep cycles and body temperature. GABA also can pass through the blood-brain barrier when administered orally. The GABA receptor sites are those affected and upregulated by benzodiazepines, barbiturates and alcohol.

"At a lecture recently, I asked people if they knew what GABA was," Jim Poole said. "No one did. We are overly reliant on stimulants for productivity, when we should better understand how key neurotransmitters such as GABA help us rest, restore and perform at maximum efficiency."

L-Theanine is a non-protein amino acid found in tea plants. It supports the formation of GABA and promotes a general calming effect. The natural effects of L-Theanine include stimulating the production of alpha brain waves, protecting and restoring the brain, inducing deep states of relaxation, and upregulating GABA to increase its clinical efficacy and relaxation effect. Studies show that L-Theanine plays a role in inducing a feeling of calm[31] and well-being, much the same as meditation, massage or aromatherapy.

These ingredients work synergistically together, along with the formula's other nutrients, to open up the GABA receptors in your brain. By doing so, they interrupt the fight-or-flight adrenaline response and begin relaxing the brain and body.

The NuCalm proprietary orthomolecular formula was developed and engineered over several years, and is only available to NuCalm users. The formula includes structured nutrient-sourced building blocks that rapidly enter the brain and convert to powerful messengers, which interrupt the body's stress response and maximize the natural relaxation response.

All of the nutrients contained in the NuCalm dietary supplements are generally recognized as safe by the FDA, which regulates them. The nutrients all have been tested for allergies and sensitivities and will not counteract or interfere with any medications or dietary restrictions.

As an alternative to the NuCalm dietary supplements, Dr. Holloway and Solace Lifesciences worked together over a period of years to develop the NuCalm Calming Cream®. This cream is also a proprietary formulation, and topically delivers the same key amino acids to balance mood and promote relaxation. Both the NuCalm dietary supplement formula and the NuCalm Calming Cream provide the same degree of benefit, offering NuCalm users two convenient options.

Note: The NuCalm dietary supplement formula may be contraindicated for pregnant and nursing women. The same warning applies for the NuCalm Calming Cream because research is insufficient to determine whether pregnant and nursing women should use it. You should always inform your doctor of any nutritional supplements you may be using.

Component Four: Light Blocking

Light blocking, with an eye mask or other means, is the final component of the NuCalm technology. Darkness reduces stimulation of the optic nerve, resulting in an immediate increase of up to 30 percent of alpha waves in the visual cortex of the brain. This enhances and further maintains the deep relaxation response that NuCalm delivers. People who may be prone to feelings of claustrophobia may choose to use dark glasses or simply shut their eyes

In considering these four NuCalm components, it's important to realize that what makes this technology unique is how each part works synergistically with each of the others. This is why NuCalm, as mentioned at the start of this chapter, is the first and only patented system in the world for balancing and maintaining the health of the human autonomic nervous system.

One expert who has tested NuCalm is Dr. Marom Bikson, co-director of neural engineering at The City College of New York and the New York Center for Biomedical Engineering. He is a recognized leader in the research and development of medical devices, including biosensors, drug delivery technologies and electrotherapy devices for neurological disorders.

Additionally, he is an acknowledged expert in medical device safety, encompassing electrical hazards, heating damage, safe stimulation protocols and electroporation. A technique involving the application of an electrical field to cells, electroporation increases cell membrane permeability to allow chemicals, drugs or other substances to enter the cell when they would not otherwise.

Dr. Bikson is an expert on the neuronal networks underlying normal brain function, including the role of the brain's bioelectric fields. He is developing new treatments for neurological diseases, such as epilepsy and depression.

In his initial study of NuCalm, Dr. Bikson used state of the art Finite Element Method stimulations on an MRI-derived model of an adult male's head. Within a few weeks of conducting his research, Dr. Bikson called to share his preliminary findings with Jim Poole.

"You are probably already aware of this," he said, "but your system works."

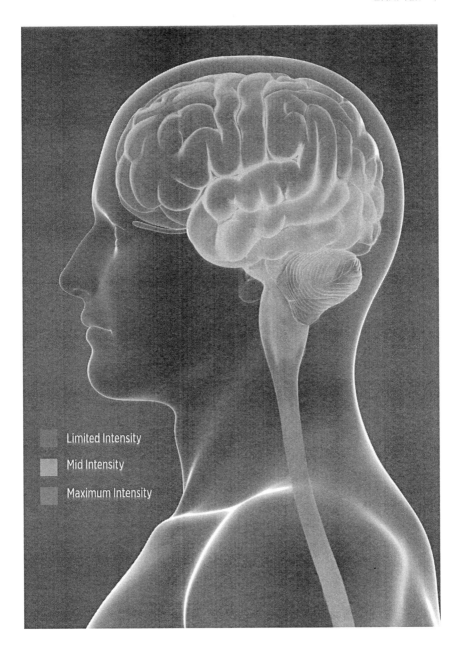

While NuCalm's effects reach the entire brain, it's maximum intensity is in the deep midbrain, the temporal cortex, the cerebellum and the brain stem. This MRI-derived model was used to illustrate research into NuCalm's efficacy by Dr. Marom Bikson, a leading expert on medical devices and their safety, the function of neuronal networks and new treatments for neurological diseases, as well as electroporation, an element of NuCalm's synergistic interactions.

NuCalm's effectiveness lies in its rapid, predictable and verifiable ability to neutralize acute stress episodes, while simultaneously balancing the autonomic nervous system for everyone who uses it. NuCalm achieves these benefits by using the brain's two communication channels: the chemical and the electrical. Within the chemical channel, CES and the NuCalm dietary supplement formula, or NuCalm Calming Cream, work together to neutralize the chemistry of the body's stress response, controlled by the HPA axis. Within the electrical channel, the NuCalm neuroacoustic software paces and entrains brain wave function, shifting from beta or high beta ranges down to the restorative alpha-theta range.

Asked about the relative importance of NuCalm's components, Dr. Holloway said:

"What I tell people is, if we could pare each component off, the neuroacoustic software provides 30 percent of the benefits, and perhaps even a bit more, while the CES and the dietary supplement formula, or calming cream, each provide another 30 percent, and then the light-blocking eye mask provides an added bonus.

"In developing NuCalm, my team and I pulled every component apart. We tested people using a single component, double components, triple components, and all of the components together. We had to do all of that to demonstrate and prove, in our patent application, that

The Sympathetic Nervous System

FUNCTIONS:

defends the body against attack: **fight or flight**
elevates blood pressure, blood sugar and body heat

REGULATES:

brain, muscles, the thyroid and adrenal glands
insulin, cortisol and thyroid hormones

ASSOCIATED EMOTIONS:

will, anger, aggression, fear, guilt and sorrow

it is the integrative effect of all four components together that makes NuCalm unique. The patent examiner we worked with challenged us on this, and because of that, all of the original research and testing that I had done had to be replicated independently, which it was, including at Harvard University. The results proved my thesis. We went through some really big hurdles, because I think the examiner couldn't quite believe it, but we prevailed."

Improving Parasympathetic Function

As you learned in Chapter 2, your body's autonomic nervous system controls and regulates homeostasis, and oversees the health and activity of bodily functions such as heart rate, blood pressure and digestion. It is comprised of two branches, the sympathetic nervous system and the parasympathetic nervous system.

The parasympathetic nervous system has a particularly important role in how and why NuCalm provides its many benefits. This is due to the difference between the parasympathetic nervous system and the sympathetic nervous system.

Your body relies on the sympathetic nervous system to maintain its defense and survival. When your autonomic nervous system is in dominant sympathetic mode, your body shifts into a fight-or-flight

The Parasympathetic Nervous System

FUNCTIONS:

heals, regenerates and nourishes the body: **rest and recovery**
activates digestion, elimination and immune function

REGULATES:

liver, kidneys, pancreas, spleen, stomach, small intestines and colon
parathyroid hormone and bile, pancreatic and digestive enzymes

ASSOCIATED EMOTIONS:

contentment, gratitude, calm and relaxation

response, diverting its energy to defend itself against threats, whether real or perceived. This is all well and good in the face of emergencies and threats to your health, such as invading disease pathogens.

However, if sympathetic dominance is maintained indefinitely, which is what happens with chronic stress, this diversion of energy deprives cells, tissues and organs. Eventually, this leaves you in a depleted, weakened state.

The parasympathetic system, by contrast, is devoted to nourishing, healing and rebuilding the body. When actively dominant, it stimulates and enhances immune function, circulation, digestion and overall gastrointestinal function. It improves functioning of the liver, stomach, pancreas and intestines. It also lowers heart rate and blood pressure levels, while increasing production of endorphins, your body's "feel good" hormones.

Only when your body is in a state of parasympathetic dominance are you able to achieve deep levels of rest and recuperation. Achieving and maintaining a healthy parasympathetic state is essential for healing on both the physical and mental-emotional levels of your being. Parasympathetic dominance enables you to be more relaxed, content and fully present in the moment. You are able to meet and respond to daily life challenges both calmly and more energetically.

Unfortunately, due to stress and autonomic nervous system imbalance, most people today find themselves primarily in a state of sympathetic nervous system dominance.

The Vagus Nerve and Heart Rate Variability

The principal pathway that nerve impulses and signals use to travel from the parasympathetic nervous system is the vagus nerve. It originates in the medulla oblongata, a part of the brainstem, and extends all the way down to the colon, supplying parasympathetic nerve fibers to organs through which it travels, except for the adrenal glands. This means that the vagus nerve not only controls various skeletal muscles, it regulates the resting state or homeostasis of most of your body's internal organs and the tasks they perform, including heart rate, respiration and gastrointestinal peristalsis. It also plays a role in vision, hearing and speech.

The vagus nerve and the parasympathetic nervous system are so closely interrelated that vagus nerve activity (vagal tone) and functionality provide a clear indication of the overall activity of the entire parasympathetic nervous system. This is especially true with regard to the influence vagal tone has on your heart rate.

Although vagal tone itself cannot be measured directly, it can be assessed by measuring other physiological processes related to the functionality of vagal tone. One of the most accurate forms of measurement is heart rate variability, which was first discussed in Chapter 2.

Also known as respiratory sinus arrhythmia, HRV refers to the difference in length of each heartbeat. For example, as previously explained, you might conclude that if a person had a pulse rate of 60 beats per minute, then each beat would last for one second. If each of the 60 beats lasted for one second, however, this would be a case of no heart rate variability, and the patient would have definite symptoms of chronic disease.

If one beat lasted for 1.0 seconds, followed by the next beat at .98 seconds, followed by the next beat at 1.02 seconds, followed by the next beat at .97 seconds, this would indicate excellent heart rate variability, and this patient would be considered quite healthy, with a positive reading on the parasympathetic nervous system.

A decrease in, or lack of, heart rate variability is a common risk factor for virtually all chronic diseases, regardless of a person's age. Research has shown that lowered HRV is associated with premature aging,[32] inflammation,[33] depression,[34] anxiety, PTSD, panic disorders,[35] decreased autonomic nerve activity, and an increased risk of sudden cardiac death after acute heart attack.[36]

Again, the more variable your heart rhythm and the more each beat is slightly different in length from the preceding beat, the healthier your autonomic nervous system is and the more parasympathetic nervous system activity you have.

Parasympathetic activity, as well as the overall functioning of the autonomic nervous system, is assessed very easily using HRV. For this test, a sensor is attached to the chest area to record the heartbeat for two minutes while the patient is lying down, and for another two minutes while the patient stands. The results are graphed, to reveal the activity of the sympathetic and parasympathetic nervous systems, with values ranging between +4 and -4 for each system.

The reason HRV testing is so effective for determining para-sympathetic nervous system activity is because your heart rate is controlled by various centers in your brainstem. One of these centers is the nucleus ambiguus, which we introduced to you in Chapter 3. The nucleus ambiguus, acting in concert with the vagus nerve, increases parasympathetic nervous system signaling to the heart. As this occurs, the heart rate slows and exhibits greater variability. So using HRV to measure heart rate enables physicians and researchers to determine overall vagal tone, and thus the level of parasympathetic nervous system activity. HRV findings can be verified through simultaneous electrocardiogram testing.

Ongoing studies, both by Dr. Holloway and independent researchers, employ both of these measurement tests, HRV and ECG. They continue to verify that the NuCalm technology provides, predictably and rapidly, a sustained increase in parasympathetic nervous system activity, which promotes and enhances the body's restorative rest and healing mechanisms. Now we will examine this research in more detail.

What Research Reveals About NuCalm

Dr. Holloway's original research, which led to the development of NuCalm, continues to be bolstered and built upon through independent testing by Solace Lifesciences and its research partners at Harvard Medical School, using algorithms developed by NASA and a cutting-edge single lead ECG HRV diagnostic-analytical tool.

Some of the world's leading scientists, academicians and clinicians currently are using the latest neuroscience equipment, diagnostic tools and mathematical models to validate NuCalm's breakthrough technology. Researchers analyze alpha-theta crossovers, ECGs, HRV, blood pulse volume, slow cortical response, neurotransmitter lab panels and galvanic skin response (the same technology used in lie detector tests).

"Alpha-theta crossovers are interesting," said Jim Poole, "because when the frequencies of the alpha and theta brain wave functions cross over each other, it is indicative of *hypnagogia,* which is a scientific term for the transitional state between wakefulness and sleep, characterized by losing a sense of time and space. Invariably, everybody who does NuCalm achieves this state, usually within 15 to 20 minutes."

In addition, since NuCalm's introduction to the field of dentistry, a variety of other objective, quantifiable techniques have been used by dentists to measure the system's efficacy, including pulse oximetry, heart rate and blood pressure readings. Another testing method, the Likert scales, is a proven and reliable questionnaire system. Dentists have used it following procedures to assess patient satisfaction with using NuCalm during treatment.

An examination of the data compiled from all the research on NuCalm makes clear why it received its unique patent, especially with regard to three of the 17 claims under that patent: first, a rapid descent into parasympathetic nervous system dominance; second, a sustained parasympathetic nervous system dominance throughout the NuCalm experience, and third, a rapid return to full lucidity.

Much of the NuCalm research was conducted and analyzed by one of the world's preeminent statistical biophysicists, Chung-Kang Peng, Ph.D., co-director of the Rey Institute for Nonlinear Dynamics in Medicine at the Beth Israel Deaconess Medical Center, a major teaching hospital at Harvard Medical School. In his research, Dr. Peng made use of the Hilbert-Huang Transform algorithm developed by NASA. The HHT algorithm provides a way to decompose a signal obtained from instantaneous frequency data. It is designed to work well for non-stationary, nonlinear data.

Dr. Peng used a single lead ECG device to capture a sensitive, accurate heart signal that was analyzed using the Kubios HRV 2.2 platform, an advanced nonlinear heart rate variability analysis software developed by the Department of Applied Physics of the University of Eastern Finland. More than 50 of these HRV platforms and ECG devices are being used currently across the United States as part of Solace Lifesciences' continuing research into the benefits of the NuCalm technology.

"This device is attached to each subject's chest and collects 250 data points per second and 15,000 data points per minute," Jim Poole said. "This data is then analyzed using complex, nonlinear dynamic, frequency-domain quantum physics to show key health indicators, such as heart rate variability, entropy and, more importantly for NuCalm, *sympatho-vagal balance*. Sympatho-vagal refers to the autonomic nervous system, with *sympatho* being the sympathetic nervous system, and *vagal* referring to the vagus nerve, which manages the autonomic nervous system and is dominant in the parasympathetic nervous system response."

Based on his own research and analysis, Dr. Peng praised the technology, saying, "On NuCalm, subjects experience a rapid decrease in heart rate and respiration rate while exhibiting an increase in vagal tonality. These biomarkers are consistent with deep meditation and illustrative of the predictable, rapid onset of the parasympathetic nervous system dominance created by NuCalm."

Much of the most recent research on NuCalm has focused on two completely different populations. The first consists of stage 4 cancer patients, who receive NuCalm treatments in conjunction with the comprehensive cancer wellness program developed by Dr. Janet Hranicky, Ph.D., co-founder of the American Health Institute and a world-renowned pioneer in the field of managing cancer with mind-body medicine approaches.

"We have been capturing data with stage 4 cancer patients since 2014," Jim Poole said. "Every three months we provide 17- to 21-day treatment plans with NuCalm to these patients and measure the health of the patients' autonomic nervous systems before and after each NuCalm session."

The second test subject population is comprised of world-class, professional athletes. "We learn the most from extremes," Jim Poole said. "That's why we've chosen these two very different test subject populations: stage 4 cancer patients and their support network, who arguably are going through one of the most difficult times in the course of their lives; and professional athletes, who arguably are the most balanced and healthiest physical specimens on the planet."

In both test populations, a baseline assessment is made of each subject's autonomic nervous system, which is monitored throughout each 30-minute NuCalm session using an ECG and the HRV analytical platform mentioned earlier. Despite the vast differences in the two populations' overall health, the baseline assessment typically reveals each test subject to be in a state of sympathetic nervous system dominance, meaning that the nervous system is locked into fight-or-flight mode.

"When you are in fight-or-flight mode all the time," Jim Poole said, "you are not getting theta brain wave function and restorative sleep, and thus, your cells are not getting the opportunity to fully cleanse themselves and maintain their cellular structure. The result is that your body is not getting the optimal healing it needs. What our research shows is that NuCalm turns off the fight-or-flight mechanism. It does this exceptionally well, rapidly and predictably. The patent office would not have awarded NuCalm the only patent in the world for systems and methods for balancing and maintaining the health of the human autonomic nervous system if NuCalm did not work."

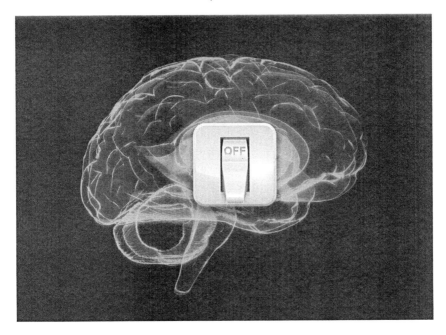

Regardless of who the test subjects are and what they are experiencing in their daily lives, the research data compiled on NuCalm verifies the patent claims. In every case, the data predictably and reliably shows a consistent pattern regarding the impact NuCalm is having on the autonomic nervous system.

Typically, within one to five minutes of initiating a NuCalm session, test subjects experience a rapid descent into parasympathetic nervous system dominance, and within 15 to 20 minutes reach a state of hypnagogic dissociation. These findings reflect the immediate and profound reduction in what are known as the *total power spectrum* and the *low frequency to high frequency (LF/HF) ratio*.

"The total power spectrum, found within the frequency-domain results of the Fast Fourier Transform algorithm, is a quantified measurement of the subject's autonomic nervous system. The tone of sympathetic nervous system is a more significant contributor to the total power spectrum," Jim Poole said. "In all cases, the total power spectrum rapidly decreased, then continued to decrease across each five-minute segment of monitoring, and this reduction was maintained throughout the entirety of each NuCalm experience."

The LF/HF ratio quantifiably assesses the balance between each test subject's sympathetic nervous system (LF) and parasympathetic nervous system (HF). Sympatho-vagal balance is imperative for professional athletes, as they need high cortisol-adrenaline sympathetic dominance to compete at extreme levels. However, just as cancer patients do, athletes also need parasympathetic nervous system dominance to optimize muscle recovery, healing and sleep quality.

During testing, both athletes and cancer patients alike consistently showed a profound decrease in the LF/HF ratio across each five-minute segment and for the duration of each NuCalm experience, indicating optimal healing. The only anomaly to the decrease in LF/HF ratio occurred when the subjects fell asleep during a NuCalm session, which elicited a spike in sympathetic nervous system activity necessary to maintain a normal heartbeat.

Another significant finding in both test populations was that many subjects using NuCalm achieved a *resonant meditator's peak*.

"This peak is achieved at the 0.1 frequency domain, which is the sweet spot for optimizing a human's biorhythm and is synonymous with 10,000 hours of monastic meditation," Jim Poole said. "When such a peak is reached, the subject's brain wave function reaches frequent alpha-theta crossovers and can maintain deep theta. The body will heal at an optimal level while also achieving maximum oxygenated blood flow.

"Most humans cannot achieve this deep level of meditation, even after years of regular practice. To achieve this level of healing by sitting down and trying to meditate, we would have to go to a monastery and learn to meditate two hours a day for over 13 years. Only then might we be able to achieve the same level of diaphragmatic breathing, relaxation and optimal healing that result from activating the parasympathetic nervous system, the heart and the lungs to pump oxygen-rich red blood cells to our entire body. That is what we see in the subjects we have tested during NuCalm sessions.

"We are not ever going to claim that using NuCalm is the same thing as meditating like a monastic monk, however.

"Meditation is learning to train your mind to let go of thoughts. NuCalm doesn't do that at all. Rather, it allows your body to heal while your mind is free to wander. Your mind does not shut off. In fact, one could argue that it accelerates and travels down very nonlinear paths because it's essentially going through the twilight zone of the alpha and theta brain wave function.

"So with NuCalm you are going to enjoy the physiological benefits achieved by deep monk-like meditation. The data we have compiled illustrates that by using the NuCalm technology you can achieve cellular homeostatic balance. You can cleanse your cells. You can oxygenate fully. And, you can achieve optimal diaphragmatic biorhythm breathing because of the way NuCalm uses neurophysiology, biochemistry and physics to mimic the healing principles of the deep cellular homeostatic sympatho-vagal balance that is synonymous with deep meditation."

Equally important is the positive, cumulative impact that occurs with repeated NuCalm use. In each case, the more each test subject experienced NuCalm, the faster and deeper the relaxation response became. This was shown by the decrease, within a shorter time each session, in their total power spectrum and LF/HF ratio.

An examination of this research data reveals other main points about NuCalm benefits. First and foremost, the data shows that it does not matter what condition a person is in when using NuCalm. "It doesn't matter what we're going through," Jim Poole said. "It doesn't matter if you are a professional athlete, or a long-haul airline pilot, or if you suffer from PTSD, depression, anxiety, addiction, stage 4 cancer or any other type of disease.

"NuCalm does the same thing to every human being that can hear, has a heart that is beating and has lungs that work. In every case, because of how NuCalm combines biochemistry, physics and neuro-physiology, it quickly put the brakes on the stress response, causing a rapid descent into parasympathetic nervous system dominance that allows the body to rest, heal, restore and rejuvenate."

Here are other key observations and results that the research data reveals:

- NuCalm predictably takes the foot off the gas pedal of the au-tonomic nervous system and provides an immediate impact of deep relaxation. It flips the switch on high cortisol and adrenaline, allowing the body to activate the brain-heart-lung connection to optimize diaphragmatic breathing, ox-ygen-rich red blood cell flow, muscle recovery and healing.

- As NuCalm provides deep relaxation throughout the body, it minimizes the negative consequences of lactic acid buildup and, most importantly, reduces inflammation that compro-mises the pace of healing.

- NuCalm provides the neurophysiology and biochemistry necessary to improve sleep quality and manage circadian rhythm dysfunction. In testing athletes, who must travel and suffer effects of frequent time zone changes, NuCalm pre-dictably reduces jet lag and manages the body's circadian rhythms, allowing for optimal performance.

- In addition to the physiological benefits identified by the research, the data shows that NuCalm enhances the mental aspects of performance and productivity. It achieves these positive effects by increasing blood flow to the midbrain, which resolves blockages and helps separate emotion from the context of daily events. This means that, instead of expending energy dwelling on challenges and possible negative outcomes, regular users of NuCalm become more resilient and calm, better able to move on, maintain their focus and achieve their goals more efficiently.

What to Expect

The NuCalm experience has been called "a massage for your mind." Just as the effects of a body massage can vary from session to session, and can produce results ranging from restful relaxation to increased energy, NuCalm experiences also will vary. The time spent in a NuCalm session also can range from 20 to 30 minutes, or up to 90 minutes or more.

Most people begin to enter deeper levels of relaxation within three to five minutes of starting the session. Their brain wave function drops from a beta state (13 to 30 Hz) to an alpha state (8 to 12 Hz), then cycles between the alpha and theta states (4 to 12 Hz).

As this occurs, they can expect to begin taking deeper breaths, because the chest cavity will move more freely as the relaxation response takes hold. The body may start to feel heavier, akin to the feeling of going to sleep. In fact, many people actually fall asleep during the session, and that's fine. It simply means that NuCalm is helping their body get the restorative rest it needs. There also may be tingling sensations in the hands or feet, because blood will be flowing to the vital organs, promoting rest and digestion.

Virtually all of the hundreds of thousands of people who have experienced a NuCalm session enter a state of deep relaxation. As they do, sympathetic nervous system activity decreases and parasympathetic nervous system activity increases.

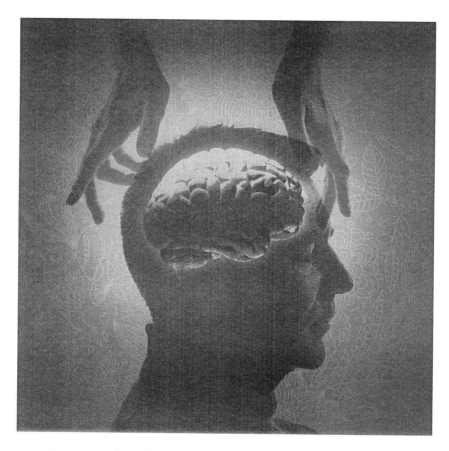

Common physiological changes include reduced muscle tension in the head and neck. Typically, the jaw slackens and opens slightly during a NuCalm session. When stressed, we often unconsciously clench the jaw, creating tension that can radiate through the rest of the body. This release of neuromuscular tension occurs because of the changes in brain waves that NuCalm creates, and because of a corresponding increase in oxygenated red blood cell flow. This release of tension can last up to several days.

Other potential physical occurrences during a NuCalm session include twitching in the fingers or toes due to neuromuscular tension release, and a sensation of gravitational pull on the face as the jaw, neck and head muscles relax completely. In some cases, especially in people whose sympathetic nervous system is highly dominant, there can be a temporary increase in heartbeat and breathing rhythms. Such sensations are typically fleeting. They are signs of the sympathetic nervous system resisting the release of control as parasympathetic activity increases.

None of the above sensations is cause for panic. They will pass as the session continues.

Although a NuCalm session sometimes causes sleep, conversely, it also can result in heightened mental acuity and awareness, akin to the "mind awake, body sleeping" state experienced by seasoned, long-term meditators. While cycling within the alpha-theta states, the mind can find surprise solutions to problems or offer new ideas and approaches to life challenges. Some people report vivid experiences similar to lucid dreaming and other related mental states.

The NuCalm technology is remarkably predictable at getting rid of stress and freeing the mind to wander. Released from worry, anxiety, fear, time constraints, expectations, self-doubt and deadlines, the mind will go where it wants to go.

Ultimately, an experience with NuCalm will be unique to each person. It depends on several physiological variables, such as the current levels of stress, body tension, rest, nourishment and any of several other factors.

In people who habitually have trouble falling asleep or who have high levels of anxiety, it can take longer to experience the brain-focused relaxation that NuCalm initiates. Instead of the usual three to five minutes, it may require 10 minutes or more to enter the alpha-theta state cycle. If that happens, simply stay with the process until the deeply relaxed state takes hold.

In someone who has difficulty relaxing and letting go, the second NuCalm experience may be more profound than the first. This response is logical, considering that the second NuCalm experience does not have to overcome curiosity, anticipatory anxiety or unknown expectations about NuCalm.

Generally, the more anxious or stressed people are, the more profound their NuCalm experience will be. Remember, each NuCalm session takes brain wave function into a 4 Hz to 12 Hz cycle. In an anxious or highly stressed person, brain waves likely are oscillating near 30 Hz, a very agitated beta state. During a NuCalm session, therefore, a more rapid or dramatic relaxation, and more beneficial effects, would occur than in people whose brain waves typically oscillate in the normal 15 Hz and 18 Hz beta levels.

One other common experience during a NuCalm session is losing track of time. Many people think their session lasted 20 to 30 minutes only to discover, once it's over, that 60 to 90 minutes have passed. This is normal, especially if they happen to fall asleep.

When using NuCalm under the supervision of a physician or dentist, the session most likely will be timed and your health practitioner will signal, perhaps with a gentle tap on the shoulder, that the session has concluded.

One question asked by NuCalm users at home is, "How will I know when my session is over?" In our experience, the answer is simple. Your body will tell you. As the session naturally runs its course, your body typically will signal that the session is coming to an end. For example, you may suddenly find yourself taking a deep breath and having the urge to open your eyes, much as you might when you awake in the morning or from a nap. Just trust the process and be aware of how you feel. By doing so, you will know when it's time to finish your session.

One of the most valuable aspects of NuCalm is its packaging of advanced neuroscience into a system that is easy to use at home. It was designed with the end user in mind, expressly to manage stress and balance the autonomic nervous system. The technology works with you and provides the opportunity for your body to enter a state of deep, health-enhancing relaxation. Once the system has resolved all your current stress and provided you with needed restoration on a cellular level, that session's job is done and you are ready to go.

With regular use, you will begin to experience heightened and sustained periods of calm, accompanied by improved physical, mental and emotional resilience. You will begin to adapt more easily to stress and daily life challenges.

Further, most people who use NuCalm consistently find that they have less need for long sessions. The physiological and psychological benefits they achieve from the system become more easily attainable and sustainable with shorter periods of dedicated practice.

These phenomena happen because NuCalm balances your autonomic nervous system and regular use keeps it healthy.

In Chapters 5 and 6, we will explore further the physical, mental-emotional and performance benefits of NuCalm. Let's end Chapter 4 with a final comment by Jim Poole, summarizing how and why NuCalm works:

"The human brain works in patterns and it is always seeking patterns. Our brains also seek shortcuts, or ways to cheat those patterns. The NuCalm technology mimics patterns that the brain identifies as deep relaxation. With NuCalm, we are not doing anything foreign; we're simply adding fuel and patterns to the brain, and the brain is taking its brain waves to deep relaxation. It doesn't matter what tools you use to evaluate NuCalm. It has an exceptional predictability and it simply does what it does. So for yourself, for your patients, for people within your businesses and, more importantly, for the friends and family that you love and hold dear to you, I encourage you to try NuCalm for yourself.

"We all need a tool to take better care of ourselves, to help with focus, to help with emotional balance, to help to be present in the moment without judgment, and to be available for our family and friends, as well as for ourselves. Thirty minutes of NuCalm will create an exceptional, productive, powerful day and a great night of restorative sleep. So give that gift to yourself, and when things get crazy or you're engaged in conflict resolution, or your emotions are dictating your decision-making, use NuCalm for 30 minutes, knowing that when you finish, you'll be performing better and people will want to be around you because of how calm and centered you are."

Chapter 5

How NuCalm Optimizes Health

We are currently living in the second age of anxiety, the first having been during and just after World War One," said NuCalm's inventor. "People are more stressed today than during the Great Depression, and they are not doing enough to manage stress and maintain healthy sleep habits.

"I think that humanity has reached a place of what I call evolutionary need. As our society continues to undergo disruptive changes and threats continue to escalate, such as terrorism, environmental degradation and the like, we can no longer rely upon the solutions of the past to manage our stress levels and meet the needs associated with our nation's, and the world's, increasing proliferation of degenerative disease."

Not only do we agree with Dr. Holloway, we know that what he says is borne out by an ever-increasing compilation of evidence and scientific data. We are living through a time when the ways and methods of the status quo are failing us, and we do need new answers and solutions to the problems we all face, especially with regard to our health and well-being.

Based on our own personal experiences using NuCalm, as well as the experiences of the hundreds of thousands of other people who have used it, we are convinced that NuCalm is at the forefront of the new technologies that are meeting the evolutionary need mentioned by Dr. Holloway.

In this chapter, we will share with you how and why regular use of NuCalm has the potential to provide significant benefits for people suffering with some of today's most serious diseases and health challenges, even though it is not, nor is it intended to be, a medical device designed to diagnose, treat or cure disease.

The main reason NuCalm offers so much promise when it comes to improving and maintaining your health is the way it predictably shuts down the stress response and promotes parasympathetic dominance. As you learned in Chapter 2, the primary daily threat to your health and performance is chronic stress, regardless of its source. Despite the body of supporting scientific evidence, skeptics may insist that the relationship between stress and disease is overemphasized. They may say that stress has always been a part of the human experience.

"Even though our Paleolithic ancestors certainly lived through scary times and experienced many stress-filled moments in their day-to-day existence as hunter-gatherers, including being attacked and chased by the predatory beasts of that time, in the evening they would take a break from that," Dr. Holloway said, explaining the flaw in such an argument. "That is to say, although the set point of their autonomic nervous systems would get very high when they were in fight-or-flight mode, the set point would not stay high once the danger passed, enabling them to shift into a relaxed, parasympathetic dominant state.

"Today, that isn't the case for most people. Although most of us do not face dangers equivalent to those of our ancestors, instead we face the struggle of coping with chronic stress, so that we are perpetually in fight-or-flight mode, even though most people are usually unconscious of being so.

"As a result, we're dealing with lots of people today who are habitually in a state of sympathetic dominance and whose autonomic set points are well outside of a healthy range. Humans need balance in their autonomic nervous system. When it is perpetually out of balance, the body will begin to break down on a cellular level, creating negative consequences.

"When we look at the signaling pathways of the brain and nervous system in people who are sympathetically dominant, we can see how their bodies are being flooded with stress hormones, as well as an increased production of *nuclear factor kappa B*, which is a genetic inflammatory switch. Science shows that when nuclear factor kappa B is not properly regulated, which is what happens when we are chronically in sympathetic nervous system dominance, it can lead to a wide range of unhealthy outcomes, including chronic inflammation and impaired immune function."

Another important way regular use of NuCalm can improve your health, according to Dr. Holloway, is how it increases nervous system *complexity*, or the resiliency so important to high-level performance.

"If you are dealing with something that lacks complexity and doesn't have all the robustness that it needs, it's not going to operate very well," he said. "I don't care what the disease state is, regardless of its cause, when we are in a state of sickness we are losing complexity. That is also what happens when we are sympathetically dominant.

"This has been demonstrated by measuring the corona around the body's cells. The corona is a little energy field around your cells that is produced by the body's electricity. In a state of health, the corona is cohesive and strong, but when it becomes affected by the body's stress responses, the corona can weaken and lose its coherency. When this happens, enzymes in and around the cells, which have a polarity and which are necessary for all of your body's processes and reactions, do not orient in the right direction. They actually get disoriented, and this lowers the body's metabolic potential.

"So any system, including the human body and brain, that is losing complexity is going toward entropy or decline. It's like a clock winding down, and you can observe it in the autonomic nervous system using the heart rate variability and ECG testing that we've done. When we use these advanced algorithms that have a nonlinear dynamic, we're getting into the area of physics. What we're observing when we look at all of the data that we are compiling is that NuCalm is increasing complexity in those persons' nervous systems."

See Chapter 4 for details of this testing by Dr. Peng at Harvard.

Another significant benefit of NuCalm is its ability to rapidly create a state consistent with deep meditation, as proven by Dr. Peng and researchers at Harvard Medical School. This finding was confirmed in January 2014, when NuCalm was approved by the Chinese national government as a "safe and efficacious intervention for stress and a replacement for meditation" under the regulations of Traditional Chinese Medicine.

In April 2016, the Chinese government took an additional step and issued a patent, as had the U.S. government in July 2015, for NuCalm and its "systems and methods for balancing and maintaining the health of the human autonomic nervous system."

Given how extensively scientists in both China and the West have studied and validated the benefits of daily meditation, NuCalm's proven and acknowledged ability to provide the same range of benefits as meditation confirms its efficacy in promoting overall health through balanced autonomic nervous system function.

The Pathways to Health and Illness

In our journey through life, it can be said that we are traveling down one of two paths. The first is the path that leads to improved and continued good health, not only physically, but also mentally, emotionally and spiritually. When we are on this path, we experience an ongoing sense of ease and passion for what we are doing, as well as abundant energy, enthusiasm and positive emotions.

Unfortunately, far too many people today are traveling down the second path, one characterized by fatigue, a lack of purpose in life, apprehensions about the future and an overall sense of tension and *dis*-ease. The longer a person travels along this pathway, the more likely some type of illness will develop.

Stress is the primary factor that determines which pathway you are traveling. The more often that you are stressed, the more your body will produce and flood itself with stress hormones; and it will do so to the same degree as the level of stress you are experiencing. In other words, the greater your level of stress, the more accelerated is your journey toward illness.

Research has repeatedly shown[1,2,3] that chronic stress leads to a torrent of subsequent effects, all of which act as further triggers for the development of disease. These stress-induced triggers, or risk factors, initiate a vicious cycle of pain, despondency and illness.

The more stressed you are:

- The worse you will sleep

- The more inflammation will negatively impact your cells, tissues and organs

- The more your body will be forced to cope with cellular breakdowns

- The more you are likely to experience a lack of energy

- The more apt you are to have negative emotions

- The more likely you will experience impaired cognitive function

- The faster you will age

- The more apt you are to develop various disease symptoms.

By contrast, the pathway to health and wellness is initiated and maintained by reducing stress and by attaining deep levels of rest and restoration each and every day.

The more you can rest and restore:

- The better you can manage your body's stress response

- The better you can sleep

- The better you can manage your body's inflammation response

- The healthier your cells will be

- The better you will feel

- The better you can think and perform

- The less you will feel your age

- The healthier you will be.

Regular use of NuCalm can create this pathway to balance, wellness and optimal health.

NuCalm and the Inflammatory Cascade

The link between stress and the body's inflammatory response is well established.[4] It is also a fact that chronic, low-grade inflammation is a contributing factor to a wide spectrum of illnesses ranging from heart disease, stroke, cancer and arthritis to gastrointestinal and respiratory problems, such as colitis, gastritis, pancreatitis and bronchitis.[5] By definition, any disease condition that ends in "itis" is at least in part due to inflammation.

Chronic inflammation also has been linked to diabetes and obesity.[6] More recently, it has been linked to brain diseases, including Alzheimer's[7] and to autoimmune diseases,[8] in which the immune system attacks parts of the body.

Many factors can trigger and maintain inflammation in the body, such as poor diet, injury, exposure to toxins, and bacterial or viral infections. Chronic stress is another often-overlooked contributing factor to inflammation.

As Dr. Holloway explained previously, chronic stress makes your body increase its production of nuclear factor kappa B, an inflammatory trigger. Stress also results in a cascade of other inflammatory triggers, such as cortisol and norepinephrine (adrenaline). Therefore, the more habitually stressed you are, the more your body is apt to be in an ongoing state of inflammation, making you far more susceptible to developing a wide range of illnesses.

As you learned in Chapter 2, we shift into a state of sympathetic nervous system dominance, or fight-or-flight mode, when we are stressed. The sympathetic nervous system and its functions certainly are necessary for achieving and maintaining outstanding health, and they play a role in helping the body recover from disease. However, it only functions optimally when balanced by regular parasympathetic nervous system dominance.

NuCalm is able to rapidly shift a person back from fight-or-flight mode into autonomic nervous system balance (homeostasis) without drugs. With regular use, NuCalm entrains the brain and nervous system to keep that balance, which makes it an extremely effective tool for stopping the inflammatory cascade of stress hormones. This helps minimize the physiological and psychological effects of inflammation itself. Dr. Holloway likens this process to successfully walking across a balance beam.

"Life and health are both akin to walking a balance beam," he said. "As we do so, there will always be some degree of oscillation, if you will. That is what makes homeostasis possible. However, many people today are widely oscillating in dramatic, unhealthy arcs. Instead of swinging in arcs of 70 degrees or more, we want to stay within a 15 to 20 degree of oscillation. This is what regular use of the NuCalm technology enables us to do, more easily than most of us are able to do on our own."

When chronic stress upsets this balance beam walk, the ensuing inflammatory cascade impairs the body's immune function. Stress overly activates the sympathetic nervous system, which then floods the body with stress hormones. These hormones can drastically impair the activity of immune cells. These include white blood cells and lymphocytes, which are a class of white blood cells that includes B cells, T cells and natural killer (NK) cells. These play a critical role in recognizing, attacking and eliminating cancer cells before they have the opportunity to clump together to form tumors.[9,10]

Stress hormones, over time, can shrink the thymus gland,[11] which acts as the immune system's master gland. Moreover, chronic stress can contribute to hormonal imbalances, particularly hormones produced by the adrenal, pituitary and thyroid glands,[12] thus creating further negative effects on the immune system. The result can be an increased susceptibility to infections and a greater risk of diseases caused by suppressed immunity.

Based on these factors, you can understand why NuCalm potentially can provide a wide range of health benefits, both directly and indirectly, given its proven ability to rapidly interrupt the stress response and naturally relax both the body and the brain.

In the remainder of this chapter, we will examine some of the most common and serious health issues for which NuCalm potentially provides benefits, and share with you real case histories of NuCalm's positive effects on people coping with a variety of challenges.

Addiction, Anxiety, Depression and PTSD

In Chapter 3, you learned that Dr. Holloway's original impetus in his multiyear journey toward inventing NuCalm was his determination to find a more effective way to help people suffering with addiction or PTSD, as well as the anxiety and depression that are so frequently co-factors in these conditions.

"People who suffer from addiction and/or PTSD, and also those for whom anxiety and depression are a problem, are essentially stuck in sympathetic nervous system dominance," Dr. Holloway said. "It's this side of the autonomic nervous system that continues to drive the anxiety, depression, worry, addictive behaviors and so forth, and which severely limits people's problem-solving abilities. The more sympathetically driven you are, the more fear-driven you become because you're really in this fight-or-flight reactivity. This is why addiction and PTSD are such problems.

"One of the main reasons people who suffer from addiction and PTSD get so depressed is because they have restricted blood flow to the prefrontal and frontal regions of their brains. You literally cannot be free of depression and anxiety if you don't have enough blood flow in these regions of the brain. Any time that the nervous system is locked into sympathetic dominance, you have reduced blood flow. Although I never conceived of it that way when I began my journey that led me to invent NuCalm, what I ended up with was something that can improve blood flow to these brain regions, because of how NuCalm effectively conducts and enhances the health of the autonomic nervous system, due to its positive effects on the vagus nerve.

"If you look at the wiring, so to speak, of the autonomic nervous system, it is the vagus nerve that extends its 'wires' throughout your body's organs and other systems. The vagus nerve pathway is your body's super highway. When its functioning is diminished due to excitation of the sympathetic nervous system, that's when many of the symptoms occur that we all experience, such as feeling sick to our stomach or having cold, clammy hands when we speak in front of large groups. This is true, as well, of addictive behaviors and PTSD.

"It's a vicious cycle that begins with stress, which overexcites the sympathetic nervous system, which then throws the parasympathetic nervous system off balance, which then reduces blood flow to the problem-solving frontal areas of the brain, which then causes even more stress. Then the cycle repeats itself in a downward spiral of poor decision-making, poor health and so forth.

"To ultimately re-regulate the autonomic nervous system, and treat PTSD and addiction effectively, you have to be able to reset the amygdala, the part of the brain responsible for autonomic responses to fear and fear conditioning. When the amygdala is highly stimulated, it purposely shuts off the reasoning part of the brain. It says, 'Run for safety first, don't think about this.' People whose amygdala is stimulated all the time don't have full brain capacity.

"That's one of the problems with trauma. Those emergency and survival organs are chronically stimulated to a point that it doesn't feel, to the person that is traumatized, that there is anything that can help them. That's why they turn to drugs and alcohol. You can't manage these issues with opiates. We've had a phenomenal failure with that approach.

"One of my concerns is the fact that we're losing veterans to suicide in alarming numbers each and every day due to ineffective PTSD treatment. The treatment options they are being given, if they are even being treated at all, are not an effective solution for them. You've got to be able to reset the neurological wiring for these people so that they are able to come back into a place of wholeness. NuCalm helps to do that."

During his career, Dr. Holloway has worked with literally thousands of patients suffering from addictions and PTSD. In many cases, both conditions were present, along with anxiety and depression. This is not surprising, according to Dr. Holloway.

"I saw so many cases of PTSD in both the alcoholic and the drug addiction populations that I treated," he said. "There's a much, much higher incidence of child abuse, including childhood sexual abuse and other traumatic events, in families scarred by alcoholism and addiction. These types of severe traumas tend to cluster a lot more in these populations. A lot of that is because of the dysfunctional family systems that produce many of the people with addictive disease.

"Today, science is demonstrating that these traumas also can be passed down to successive generations through their genes, just as one's physical genetic makeup can predispose one to addiction. So resolving that trauma and helping people to reframe past traumatic events in a way that the events no longer have a negative pull on them is very, very important. NuCalm is very useful in that regard.

"I've worked with over 2,000 people so far who suffered from PTSD. Many of them served in the military, and many others developed PTSD from other types of experiences. PTSD is the same for everyone. It doesn't matter what theater you got it in, whether it was through assault, the military or anything else; in the brain, it's the same thing. We have found NuCalm, although it isn't always the solution, to be extremely helpful for most people with PTSD.

"There's a physics dynamic to PTSD that people haven't really thought about. When trauma occurs, in the brain it's essentially akin to what happens when you try to put 220 volts of electricity through 110 volt wiring. Your entire nervous system has to buffer itself in order to survive. It's that buffering that causes the problems with PTSD, with the traumatic memories never being metabolized.

"We've learned an awful lot about this over the years. What I was looking for during my invention process, which is what I ended up with, was a solution that was not too expensive, did not require a lot of effort, and had a predictable, positive clinical response for addiction and PTSD. And that is NuCalm."

The following case histories are only two examples of the many positive outcomes Dr. Holloway has achieved using NuCalm to help his patients deal with addiction and PTSD. Both of these patients were participants in the happy hour sessions that Dr. Holloway discussed in Chapter 3.

The first patient was a 42-year-old male, from a well-to-do family, who suffered from chronic circadian rhythm dysfunction and was a poly-substance abuser (mostly alcohol and cocaine) with co-morbid anxiety disorders. "These issues did not get addressed during his previous treatments because it was interpreted that he was simply 'drug seeking' his way through 18 consecutive treatment centers," Dr. Holloway said. Upon coming to Dr. Holloway for help, the patient used NuCalm at least five times a week for four months to manage his stress response and to reset his circadian rhythm.

"The key during withdrawal is to manage the sympathetic arousal because it dominates the brain chemistry and blood flow, which cognitively impairs thinking and drives the addictive behaviors," Dr. Holloway said. "After four months of NuCalm therapy, this gentleman achieved autonomic nervous system balance and harmony and, during the five years that I followed his progress afterward, he did not have a single relapse. Prior to coming to me he had repeatedly relapsed soon after, and even during, his previous stays at addiction treatment centers."

The second case involved a 28-year-old female addict who was a childhood victim of sexual abuse. "She had undergone years of counseling trying to cope with what had happened to her, but the counseling never reset her autonomic nervous system," Dr. Holloway said. "Every time she would experience a trigger, caused by her having been abused, she would experience a panic attack. Her mind and body would resort to drugs, in her case benzodiazepines, and alcohol for self-medicating purposes."

The woman underwent intensive outpatient care with Dr. Holloway, using NuCalm at least five times per week for two months. Dr. Holloway combined NuCalm with cognitive behavioral therapy to create new patterns in her brain and to disconnect her emotions from the context of the abuse memories, thus facilitating new processing dynamics within her brain. After that two-month period, the woman became completely clean and sober, and no longer suffered from trauma due to her childhood tragedy. Today, more than a decade later, she has remained sober and has chosen to help others by becoming a master's level alcohol and drug therapist.

Dental Procedures

Dentistry was one of the first branches of medicine to begin using the NuCalm technology. As mentioned in Chapter 1, since NuCalm first became commercially available in September 2010, more than 700,000 dental patients across five continents have experienced NuCalm with a satisfaction rate of over 95 percent.

One of the dentists who now makes NuCalm a standard part of his dental practice is Dr. David A. Little, a dental surgeon in San Antonio, Texas. "For the past six years, I have personally used NuCalm at least twice a week," he said. "It has increased my energy level and focus, and more importantly has improved how I manage stress. Clinically, I use NuCalm on every patient. For implant procedures, I often combine NuCalm with nitrous oxide. For everyone else, it's just NuCalm. In fact, if I walk into the operatory and my patient is not using NuCalm, I walk out until they are relaxing on NuCalm. I have been at this too long to endure patient anxiety. When my patients are relaxed on NuCalm, I can also relax, focus and do my best work. NuCalm will become the standard of care in dentistry."

Another leading dentist who employs NuCalm in his practice is Paul Denemark, a dental surgeon with a master's in dentistry, a diplomate of the American Board of Periodontology and past president of the Illinois Society of Dental Anesthesiology. He first began using NuCalm in 2009 during its clinical and market research phase.

"I cannot imagine doing dental surgery without NuCalm," Dr. Denemark said. "It has become my standard of care. NuCalm consistently provides an exceptionally positive experience for my patients. It allows me to relax and focus during surgery, and my patients seem to heal faster and with fewer complications. What most impresses me about NuCalm is that it is remarkably reliable and predictable. I never have to be concerned about my patient's emotional state, even for my sedation patients. NuCalm allows me to use less and get more out of sedation protocols. NuCalm is a major advancement for dental procedures."

Dr. Denemark maintains a full-time dental practice focused on periodontics and dental implant reconstruction. As a periodontist, he supports the structures of teeth, rebuilds gum and bone, remedies dental disease states and, when necessary, replaces the teeth of his patients. Before including NuCalm in his practice, Dr. Denemark said, "My typical pre-operative protocol began with me spending a tremendous amount of time gaining my patients' trust. Part of gaining their trust involves understanding not just their physical condition, but also their emotional state. Most, if not all, patients present with varying degrees of fear, anxiety and stress about a pending surgical procedure. I would often have to spend a good deal of time with them discussing their concerns and doing what I could to alleviate their fears and anxieties.

"Though my pre-operative protocol still involves spending time with my patients to gain their trust and discuss their treatment options, since I began using NuCalm, I now rely on it as a first-line modality to relax them, and I now know that they can be virtually anxiety-free within five to eight minutes. As a result, my treatment planning has changed. I schedule shorter surgical time since I no longer have to account for a lengthy set-up or post-surgical recovery period. My surgical assistants are administering NuCalm prior to surgery, so my time is spent caring for other patients during that time.

"Once NuCalm relaxation occurs, I can anesthetize my patients more quickly, and the onset of anesthesia seems to be quicker and more profound as well, probably due to the slower metabolism caused by NuCalm's relaxation response. My patients today are more cooperative and surgery can begin sooner than without NuCalm. My patient's response to local anesthesia seems to be much less of an event compared to what it was before I began using NuCalm. Patients just don't react so negatively anymore. And, since they are very relaxed, they are very receptive to all aspects of the surgical experience, which in the past was at times a lengthy and arduous task."

Just as significantly, Dr. Denemark said that his use of NuCalm with his patients also has improved his patients' recovery after surgery. "Post-surgically, I have been surprised by my findings," he said. "I have noticed that my patients are reporting less pain and swelling for nearly all of the surgical procedures I perform. My patients also tell me that they are taking either less medication or none at all, and the incidences of post-operative complications have become fewer, as well. When I call patients in the evening after surgery, they are telling me that they feel fine and are quite surprised that they are not experiencing severe pain. In many cases, they are able to get a full night's sleep and by the next day experience only minor irritations due to their surgical experience."

The following case histories illustrate that NuCalm can help accelerate patient healing following dental surgical procedures. The first case involved a 28-year-old male patient who did not receive NuCalm, which Dr. Denemark described as a typical case and typical healing results without the benefit of NuCalm treatment.

"This patient was referred to me for extraction of a tooth, followed by an immediate implant placement with bone grafting," Dr. Denemark said. "His medical history revealed no abnormalities. His tooth had significant decay and was not restorable. The procedure was a success, and his post-operative examination with me one week later demonstrated what can be expected for a normal course of healing without NuCalm. He had slight inflammation in the area around the surgical site, which was evident by the presence of erythema (redness of the surrounding gum), edema and slight hemorrhage."

The second case involved a 66-year-old woman who also required a tooth extraction. "Her tooth had a vertical fracture and fistula on the attached gum," Dr. Denemark said. "She had an unremarkable medical history, but we noted an elevated systolic blood pressure at the beginning of her appointment. Her blood pressure was 149/72. She underwent the NuCalm relaxation protocol and we extracted her tooth, followed by immediate implant placement, bone grafting and placement of sutures.

"During the surgery, we noticed that her bleeding was less than we would have normally expected, given her slightly elevated blood pressure. At the conclusion of her surgery, we again measured her blood pressure, which was 124/70. I believe this reduction was due to the effect of NuCalm in significantly reducing her dental anxiety, especially during the stress of dental surgery. One week later, we removed her remaining sutures and she was found to have significant soft tissue healing and resolution of the fistula."

The third case in involved a 47-year-old female. "She was scheduled to receive dental implants to replace three teeth after orthodontic extrusion was completed," Dr. Denemark said. "This woman had a 30-year history of smoking a pack of cigarettes a day, and had had numerous traumatic dental experiences which created a tremendous amount of anxiety about her future dental care. She was very anxious about intravenous sedation and, given her decreased lung function due to her history of smoking, my decision was to utilize NuCalm for her surgical treatment.

"The extraction of her three teeth was performed with immediate implant placement, bone grafting with resorbable barrier membranes, and stainless steel fixation tacks. Suturing also was performed. She was followed for four months prior to placement of final abutments and porcelain fused to metal restorations. I saw her again 18 days after the first surgical procedure and her healing at that time showed the impressive healing response that I believe was due to the effects of NuCalm."

Summing up his experience with NuCalm, Dr. Denemark said, "It has been my pleasure to see the beneficial results of NuCalm for my patients. I am finding that healing is improving when I use NuCalm during treatment. I am observing decreased anxiety during the surgical phase of treatment that is helping with reduced bleeding and initial healing, and extending post-operatively with reduction in pain and swelling. Because of NuCalm, I have been able to reduce the need for stronger post-operative pain medications. NuCalm is quick to surgery, surgery while feeling assured that they will have a better surgical outcome."

As the following testimonial illustrates, not only dental patients benefit from NuCalm but also the dentists themselves. Dr. Kevin Bril, a dental surgeon in Big Lake, Minnesota, said, "My NuCalm journey started a couple of years ago when I was introduced to it at the International College of Cranio-Mandibular Orthopedics conference in Arizona. The concept was explained to me in good detail and, to be quite honest, it sounded too good to be true. I thought it was gimmicky and did not believe it could achieve what the presenters were claiming, but I was intrigued enough to give it a try. I laid out by the pool and was placed on NuCalm.

"During the first few minutes I remember thinking to myself, 'I knew this wasn't going to work.' The music was soothing but I didn't feel any different. As I sat there, I realized that the music I was listening to was not the same anymore. I thought to myself, 'What is going on?' I was tapped on the shoulder a short time later. I took off the headphones and eye mask, and talked with someone from the company. I felt so relaxed and rested, it was kind of unbelievable. He asked me how long I thought I was on NuCalm. I guessed maybe 25 to 30 minutes. Turns out it was one hour and fifteen minutes later. I was sold after that. I bought two systems that day.

"This has had a profound effect on my practice, and the majority of people that I place on NuCalm absolutely love it. They feel better when they leave and are more relaxed while I work on them. It makes for a much more enjoyable working atmosphere when the patient has a great experience in my dental chair.

"I am a 33-year-old dentist who owns a business, has two kids under the age of three and travels a lot for continuing education. To put it kindly, my world is filled with a ton of stress. I spend 40 hours a week treating patients who are less than thrilled to see the dentist. After that, I have to run the business side of the office and manage my team. Then I go home to the chaos of two young children. The last

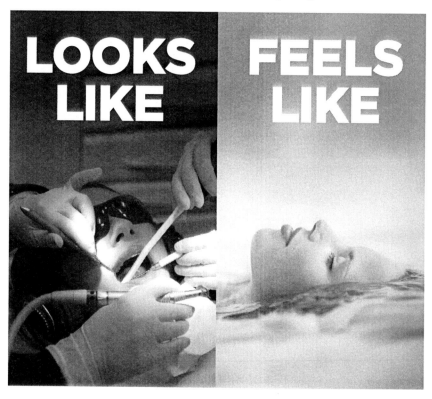

thing I want to do when coming home is to be so irritable that my kids and wife don't want to be around me.

"How do I mitigate that stress? I use NuCalm three to four times every week to recharge my batteries. I look at it as a reset button. I am able to calmly handle the stresses in my life without allowing them to turn my world upside down. My wife can always tell when I have not used NuCalm in a while. The irritability always shows through. Family life is much easier when our stress level is low. I have also noticed that when I use NuCalm I always experience increased energy and increased focus, and I sleep much better at night. The NuCalm technology really has been a game changer for my practice, my patients and my family."

Another dentist who has experienced NuCalm's many benefits firsthand is Dr. Druian, the London dental surgeon mentioned in Chapter 1. He said, "NuCalm really is one of society's biggest secrets. It has helped so many of my patients to quickly achieve deep relaxation and virtually eliminate dental-related anxiety. But, more importantly, it has made life so much easier for myself, for my hygienists and for my team. In a dental practice, NuCalm is a game changer, period.

"I must tell you how NuCalm has helped me on two levels personally. I travel from my home in London to the U.S. five or six times a year, sometimes more often. I NuCalm on the flight. This not only deeply relaxes me, but the headphones block out the sound of the engines and I experience great benefits. I can get off the plane, whether it is in America or back in the U.K., and get straight down to work. No jet lag. Nothing. My team at home can never believe it when I get off a trans-Atlantic flight, go home to shower and change, and go straight to the dental office. I have energy and enthusiasm. I will probably NuCalm that night before bed, too. It's wonderful.

"However, it's on another level that NuCalm is even more amazing. I am an insomniac. I worry about everything. If I have a very busy day the next day, I can't sleep because I worry. If my practice is going through a slow period, I worry. I even worry that I can't sleep and that I'm going to be tired the next day. It's a self-fulfilling prophecy because I'm a wreck the next day. Now, I am different because of NuCalm. If I'm up at 2 a.m., I will NuCalm for two to three hours.

By doing so, I know my brain is resting, so all is well. I get up at the normal time and carry out a great day's work with enthusiasm and no stress. I feel relaxed and rested, and I am filled with good humor.

"Overall, you have no idea what this has done for me. I even have one or two team members starting to NuCalm at home on a regular basis. I just want to thank Dr. Holloway and the Solace Lifesciences team for bringing this amazing technology to the world. It's changed my life and I can't imagine not having it." (NuCalm's benefits related to both jet lag and sleep issues are found later in this chapter.)

Cancer

Cancer is predicted to overtake heart disease as our nation's No. 1 killer. In 1975, cancer deaths were about half that of deaths related to heart disease. By 2013, cancer and heart disease each accounted for some 23% of total deaths in the U.S.[13] Current estimates are that almost one in every two men will develop some type of cancer during his lifetime, as well more than one-third of all women.[14] While early detection of cancer has improved, true survival rates are a mixed bag[15] despite the billions of dollars spent on cancer research[16,17] since President Nixon declared war on cancer in 1971.

However, the field of *psychoneuroimmunology,* or PNI, is one area of research that is showing great potential in the fight against cancer. PNI continues to identify the mental, psychospiritual and emotional factors that can predispose people to develop cancer, as well as identify what factors can improve cancer patient outcomes.

This branch of science contends that the way patients cope with stress and the effect stress has on the autonomic nervous system, with its cascade of reactions like chronic inflammation, have a tremendous impact on the survival of cancer cells.[18]

"When you look at cancer studies with heart rate variability testing, you will find that there is always a shift in the autonomic nervous system," Dr. Holloway said. "Cancer isn't something you catch. Cancer develops when your body's immune system is not taking care of rogue cells.

"Everybody develops cancer cells every day, but your oncogene (a mutation of a gene involved in normal cell growth) sends in a little protein message that tells the cancer cells to die. This is called programmed cell death, or *apoptosis*. It's when this system, which is part of the immune system, is not working that you can end up with cancer.

"That's why you see lots of people who have endured trauma and chronic stress in their lives ending up with cancer, as well as autoimmune diseases. So the ability to have a tool like NuCalm that mitigates stress, and balances and enriches the health of the autonomic nervous system, which is exactly what our patent proves that NuCalm does, is very important, especially for cancer patients."

Solace LifeScience's ongoing research project with stage 4 cancer patients started in 2014 as a collaboration with Dr. Peng of Harvard and Dr. Hranicky of the American Health Institute. Chapter 4 details their credentials, as well as the advanced equipment and methodologies used by Dr. Peng to measure NuCalm's impact on the autonomic nervous system and sympatho-vagal balance. What follows are more details about the research results.

Under Dr. Hranicky's direction, stage 4 cancer patients are using NuCalm to help them effectively manage midbrain stress and reduce overstimulation of the sympathetic nervous system. This helps alleviate nausea, improve sleep quality and reduce the impaired cognitive function caused by chemotherapy, sometimes called chemo brain. The data collected from these patients indicates that effective stress management through repeated NuCalm use can improve immune function and enhance psychoneuroendocrine (mind/nervous system/hormone) regulation of the immune system.

During this research, each cancer patient sits comfortably for a 15-minute baseline assessment of current stress levels and of the patient's autonomic nervous system. Then, the patient receives a NuCalm session for as long as needed (a minimum of 30 minutes for the research project) while resting in a comfortable chair with a blanket. Data points are captured every second throughout the session. The following illustration is from one of the cancer patients in this ongoing study and reflects the patient's first NuCalm experience, beginning with the baseline assessment.

As shown in the adjacent illustration, the LF/HF ratio quantifiably illustrates the balance of the sympathetic nervous system (LF) and the parasympathetic nervous system (HF). Sympatho-vagal balance is important for people battling disease, such as stage 4 cancer, because they must be able to turn off the adrenaline response so that the body can restore, recover and heal. In all of the research conducted thus far, cancer patients have consistently shown a profound decrease in the LF/HF ratio across each five-minute segment of observation and testing, as well as across the duration of each NuCalm experience, indicating an optimal healing zone of deep, highly oxygenated respiration.[15]

The only anomaly to the decrease in LF/HF ratio has happened when the subjects fell asleep during a session, which elicited a spike in sympathetic nervous system activity in order for the body to maintain its normal heartbeat. When the cancer patients fell asleep during their respective NuCalm experiences, the sleep activity did not last long, typically between one and four minutes. They came up from sleep and continued experiencing the deep relaxation associated with theta brain wave function.

The research data showed a consistent pattern regarding NuCalm's impact on the autonomic nervous system, a finding true for every cancer patient tested with NuCalm. Within one to five minutes of starting a session, each of them experienced a rapid descent into parasympathetic nervous system dominance and hypnogogic dissociation, reflected by the immediate and profound reduction in the total power spectrum and the LF/HF ratio.

As a brief review of the explanation in Chapter 4, the total power spectrum is within the frequency-domain results of the Fast Fourier Transform algorithm used for analyzing test results. The total power spectrum is a quantified measure of both parts of the patient's autonomic nervous system, with the sympathetic tone as a more significant contributor.

In this illustration, the patient's total power spectrum rapidly decreased, continued to decrease across each five-minute segment, and maintained reduction throughout the entirety of the NuCalm session. The total power spectrum decreased by 16 percent in the first five minutes and by 92 percent after 25 minutes on NuCalm.

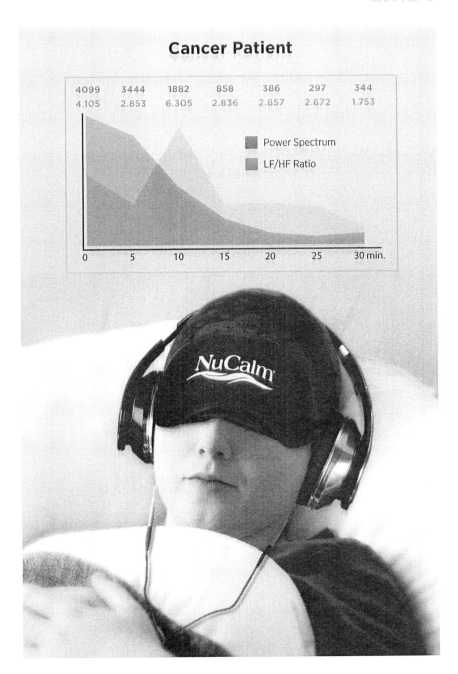

Cancer Patient

4099	3444	1882	858	386	297	344
4.105	2.853	6.305	2.836	2.857	2.672	1.753

Power Spectrum

LF/HF Ratio

Stage IV cancer patients tested with NuCalm consistently showed rapid descent into parasympathetic dominance with strong drops in the total power spectrum and LF/HF ratios. This patient's TPS dropped 92 percent during her NuCalm session. Her LF/HF spiked when she fell asleep, then continued decreasing.

Notably, this patient achieved a resonant meditator's peak while experiencing NuCalm. Most humans cannot achieve this level of meditation. This peak occurs at the 0.1 frequency domain and, as explained by Jim Poole in Chapter 4, is synonymous with 10,000 hours of monastic meditation. A 0.1 frequency domain is calculated by dividing six breaths by 60 seconds. Six breaths per minute produces the ideal for breathing biorhythms and for coherent functioning in the human body.[19] At this peak, brain wave function reaches frequent alpha-theta crossovers and can maintain a deep theta state, where the body can heal most effectively and can achieve maximum oxygenated blood flow.

Although NuCalm does not create meditation per se, it synergistically uses neurophysiology, biochemistry and physics to mimic the healing state of deep cellular homeostasis and sympatho-vagal balance, which is equivalent to deep meditation.

All of the tested cancer patients showed a cumulative positive effect with repeated NuCalm usage. The more the subjects experienced NuCalm, the faster and deeper was their relaxation response, as indicated by the faster decrease in the total power spectrum and the LF/HF ratio over a shorter time.

Commenting on her research using NuCalm with cancer patients, Dr. Hranicky said, "My background is in the field of psycho-neuroimmunology and cancer. For 35 years, I have been involved in international work that addresses the mind-body aspects of healing. I have been incorporating the NuCalm technology as part of my Comprehensive Cancer Wellness Program because of its proven ability to remediate stress at the midbrain level without drugs or psychotherapeutic intervention.

"There is an extensive body of research in the literature that shows a strong correlation between stress, psychological factors and cancer. A great deal of evidence exists linking an individual's stress response to not only the development and course of cancer but, just as importantly, to their response to treatment as well.

"It is my belief that the NuCalm technology will be an important adjunctive therapy in the future, to be incorporated with standard medical treatment in the intervention of cancer. The preliminary results of our pilot research study, using NuCalm for eight to 12 sessions over a three-week period in a cancer patient population, are indicating a definite impact on strengthening the parasympathetic nervous system and downregulating stress physiology as evidenced by pre- and post-testing with heart rate variability.

"I wrote a psychological theory of cancer called the 'Pleasure-Freeze Theory' in which I described a third response to stress that can occur, in addition to the fight-or-flight mechanism that is widely known. While experiencing a state of emotional pleasure-comfort, the parasympathetic nervous system is engaged, and a person's body experiences chemical changes which create a state of physical ease, mixed with normal levels of excitement (unfolding growth potential). Optimal physical health occurs in this state.

"When a person's sources of pleasure are blocked, or are perceived as blocked, the natural 'movement toward' process becomes unavailable. The natural pursuit of emotional pleasure will not occur, and the person will instead 'freeze' that desire rather than discharging it. This 'pleasure-freeze' sets up a physical and emotional state of tension that can adversely affect our health.

"NuCalm naturally relaxes the body within minutes, which allows the limbic area of the brain to experience a state of perceived safety and comfort that engages and triggers a parasympathetic response, and the chemical changes physiologically connected with it. Our cognitive behavioral responses are important in the learned relaxation response.

"However, it is virtually impossible for the frontal cortex to convince the limbic brain that it is safe to relax if there is a long-standing learned stress response that has been programmed, such as what we see with the pleasure-freeze, and which creates a neuro-association that pleasure and pain are connected.

"NuCalm provides the experience of deep relaxation, coupled with emotional safety, that allows the learned pleasure-freeze stress response, which I have seen clinically with cancer patients, to be interrupted so that a new and healthier response can be habituated.

"Neuronal coherence requires the circuitry between the limbic brain and the frontal cortex to be aligned. NuCalm works on the neuronal pathways linking the circuitry between thoughts and primitive emotions that have been wired for survival responses.

"In addition, research has shown that the pituitary gland is not only the master gland of the body, but it also sends out signals that promote regeneration of the other major glands and organs of the body. This process appears to involve growth hormone. Thus, stimulating the pituitary gland can stimulate regeneration throughout the body.

"The pituitary gland, being part of the limbic system, is closely associated with emotions. This book's co-author, my husband Dr. Michael Galitzer, in his research in bio-energetic medicine, showed in 1993 that the state of emotional pleasure stimulates the pituitary gland. NuCalm's technology has been shown to induce predictable states, not only of deep relaxation, but also of associated emotional pleasure, that seem to be linked to the parasympathetic nervous system becoming strengthened.

"It can be hypothesized that there is a direct link between deep relaxation and pleasure and the process of self-regeneration," Dr. Hranicky said. "This concept provides the basis for exciting future research in the area of integrating new technologies, such as NuCalm, to look at its impact on resiliency training and on stimulating the pituitary gland. Inducing regular states of deep relaxation and pleasure or comfort to attain coherency in the brain, necessary for regulating balance and homeostasis for health, is of particular importance for patients dealing with cancer and other potentially life-threatening diseases."

What follows are testimonials from cancer patients, their loved ones and their caregivers, for whom regular use of NuCalm has made a positive difference.

The first testimonial comes from Rob O., a leader of a nonprofit organization that runs a camp for terminally ill children and their families. "I want to share some experiences I've witnessed firsthand regarding the use of NuCalm," he said. "I'm personally very involved in a nonprofit organization with the mission of bringing the healing power of laughter to seriously ill children. For the past eight years, we have held dozens of illness-specific camps, attended by thousands of children. These camps are all operated under the supervision of medical professionals, and are completely free of charge to the children and their families.

"There is a measurable and defined increase in traits such as independence, strength, confidence and courage, which parents report that these young kids gain by spending time at our camps with us. We also conduct outreach programs at hospitals to provide camp activities to kids who are not able to get away to a camp.

"My story begins with a dear personal friend who introduced me to NuCalm. Upon experiencing the relaxing effects that NuCalm offers, I began to think, 'What if I could bring the many benefits of NuCalm to these children and their families?' I made some inquiries and, lo and behold, NuCalm was all for supporting this. I soon received six of them, all donated by Jim Poole, the CEO of NuCalm.

"We recently had an Oncology Family Retreat where we implemented the use of NuCalm. It was a smashing hit! Everyone was able to try it out, and the results were immediate. Each day a different family would be supplied with NuCalm. What surprised most parents was just how much their kids loved the music, and how eager they were to use NuCalm during siesta time and at night. The benefits were also clearly obvious, as they stated their children slept better and had less fatigue during the day.

"I want to thank NuCalm, and Jim Poole especially, for sharing this terrific technology with our families. I can't begin to imagine what a parent must feel, and deal with, on a daily basis when your child has a serious illness like cancer, but it does make me feel good to know that for those few special days, NuCalm made their lives just a little better.

"To conclude, here is a quote from a mother who attended the camp in July. 'Our child is very sick and has suffered so terribly. We were blessed to attend this amazing camp this week and use NuCalm. I want to personally thank you for reaching out to us in this way. It was a blessing. You have no idea how much hope you've given our family, especially our daughter. What a blessing you are. Keep up the good work!'"

The next testimonial comes from a 73-year-old woman, who wrote, "I am a thyroid cancer survivor, as well as having an assortment of other medical problems, some of which no one seems to be able to figure out. When I started using NuCalm about eight months ago, it felt like it took me a bit to relax and get my mind to slow down and then I would 'sleep' for about 45 minutes. After just a few NuCalm experiences, I noticed I felt generally calmer and things didn't seem to bother me as much as they used to.

"As I continued to use NuCalm, my body almost asked for the rest in the early afternoon, which quickly became my favorite time to NuCalm. Now I go into my meditative state quickly and wake happy and energized in approximately 25 minutes. My body is more alert, better balanced both physically and mentally, and I have added pizzazz.

"Most of the time my ears used to ring and I was diagnosed with tinnitus. After about three months of regular NuCalm relaxation, I suddenly realized the ringing was gone. I have also not experienced a single attack of vertigo since I began using NuCalm. The neuropathy I lived with for years is gone, as well, and my inflammatory myopathy disorders have lessened significantly.

"I attribute this to regular relaxation and rejuvenation through NuCalm. I am not taking any medications for these frustrations. My list of unsolved medical concerns is extensive and I do believe this system has given me the strength and opportunity to become a stronger woman. NuCalm has inspired me and I can feel an extra bounce in my being, at the age of 73. Thank you, thank you, thank you."

The next two testimonials come from Jackie and her husband Greg, and illustrate how regular NuCalm use has helped both of them cope better with Jackie's cancer diagnosis, as well as other stressful life issues.

We begin with Jackie, who wrote, "NuCalm is magical! It allowed me to shoulder a diagnosis of stage 4 incurable metastatic cancer. Last year I had bilateral cobalt-chrome rods placed in my spine to support two vertebrae lost to tumor growth. A 17-inch scar marked the seven-bone fusion that was performed in order for me to be able to walk again. When I learned that the rods were bilaterally broken less than ten months post-surgery, I had instant anxiety about having to endure another nine-hour-long procedure and the recovery. I was one month away from seeing our kids graduate high school and middle school. I was a wreck! NuCalm quickly defused my panic, which allowed me to hear my orthopedic surgeon's advice without drama and emotion obscuring the plan of action.

"In the same week, my 84-year-old mom suffered a stroke. With NuCalm, I was able to direct my attention to her needs. I was also

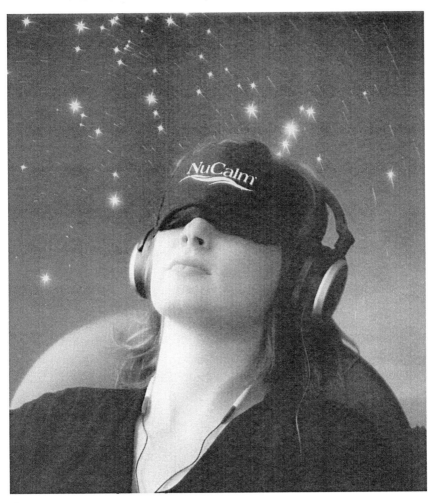

able to administer NuCalm on my mother during her admittance. While she utilized NuCalm in the ER, I observed her heart rate, pulse and breathing relax while she was connected to the monitors. In my condition, I knew I couldn't care for her, yet because of NuCalm, this was another added stress that seemed to wash away as I watched her regain speech and recover from right side paralysis. I now use NuCalm to manage daily stress.

"We have a freshman in college, a daughter beginning high school, aging parents and me living with broken rods which did not need to be removed after all because my body is healing. NuCalm has proven effective for all of life's transitions, pain, anxiety and sleep issues."

Jackie's husband Greg added, "April 15, 2014: 'Stage 4 incurable metastatic cancer to your spine' were the words delivered to Jackie and me at 11:34 a.m. Shock! Fear! Denial! It's difficult to process such information by any measure. An immediate, unavoidable stress consumes you entirely, to be sure. There is no way around it, and denial is only a short-term delay. Eventually such a statement is going hit you hard. Either deal with it or die. No matter how you slice it. No matter who you are. The only winning strategy is one grounded in taking personal responsibility for your health.

"What ensued for Jackie and myself is what could be described as a tsunami of stress. April 15, 2014, tax day, became day one of 218 consecutive 14-hour days of me taking over all duties and responsibilities in our home and family. We all know that the management of family, home and business can be daunting. Now, heap onto that pile the 24-hour care of someone who is immobile and incapable of performing the simplest of tasks. Heap onto that the task of learning everything that has been discovered in the treatment of cancer. Then add a dash of discovery revealing the darker side of medicine as shown illuminated by the light of holistic health care.

"If you manage to maintain clarity through this process, then try explaining your findings to friends and family, enlightening them on the position that you know better than the medical doctors and you're going to take a pass on those treatment protocols, and instead you'll heal yourself naturally with nutrition and other holistic modalities.

Let me know how that goes. Then heap onto that pile, now that you've decided to go holistic, the new tasks of creating and sourcing the raw materials that you need to support your new lifestyle choice. You guessed it; I became a farmer on April 16th.

"Some 218 plus days later, and owing to a strength of will unmatched in the universe, Jackie and I are presented with a gift. The gift that comes to all who endure...an introduction to remarkable people, doing remarkable things and possessing a remarkable technology called NuCalm.

"The hard work is in the past and remains only a distant memory. The struggle, heartbreak, pain, stress and suffering that Jackie and I have endured is a thing of the past. What remains is the reward. What remains is NuCalm. NuCalm provides me with balance, clarity, positive energy, an ability to manage many things at once, and a quality of sleep I've never before experienced as an adult. NuCalm has changed our lives! This technology has dramatically reduced the stress in Jackie's life, allowing her immune system to fight cancer as it was designed to do, and NuCalm has given me the edge that I need to support that effort."

We conclude this section by sharing the case history of a patient for whom regular NuCalm use helped result in a complete recovery from cancer. This patient is a close personal friend of David Poole, Solace Lifesciences' executive vice president of marketing. Mike T. was diagnosed with a combination of testicular and abdominal cancer.

"Mike was in trouble," David Poole said. "Knowing what I do about stress and cancer, I made sure he had NuCalm to help him get through the challenging ordeal he faced. He used it regularly, and as a result, despite undergoing a rigorous treatment protocol with chemotherapy, he was able to go about his daily life without the need to miss work, nor did he experience the degree of fatigue and other side effects that are commonly experienced during chemotherapy treatments.

"In fact, during his treatment, he gained 12 pounds, and his blood work proved to be an anomaly, too, because it was so healthy. His doctors were baffled by that. I'm happy to report that today he is cancer-free and doing quite well, and he continues to use NuCalm as part of his overall health maintenance routine because of how it helped him journey through cancer and back to good health."

Heart Disease

The incidence of heart disease has remained high, keeping its ranking as No. 1 killer in the United States, even though survival rates have increased.[20] Once a condition that primarily targeted men, today heart disease affects women at almost the same rate as men. In fact, one in four deaths each year among women in the U.S. now are caused by heart disease.[21] (We share more statistics related to heart disease in Chapter 2.)

Further compounding these problems is the incidence of high blood pressure (hypertension) among Americans today. High blood pressure is a major risk factor for heart disease, including heart attack and stroke. Despite the need to control blood pressure levels, approximately one-third of all American adults have high blood pressure, including many people in their early 20s. Additionally, another third of all Americans suffer from pre-hypertension, meaning they are at risk for developing high blood pressure. Most alarmingly, more than 20 percent of people with high blood pressure are unaware of their condition because high blood pressure is all too often undiagnosed.[22]

The science to determine what causes heart disease continues to evolve. As it does, what were once accepted as primary risk factors are being re-evaluated as perhaps being secondary issues. Beginning in the 1950s, the main cause of heart disease was claimed to be high cholesterol levels. As a result, cholesterol-rich and high-fat foods were demonized. Doctors warned their patients away from such foods. Cholesterol-lowering drugs, especially statins, were prescribed widely, not only to patients with heart disease, but also as a preventive measure.

Today, a growing body of scientific evidence challenges these approaches. Researchers are finding that high fat and high cholesterol foods are not the problem, but sugar and a preponderance of carbohydrate foods in the diet.[23] Statin drugs, though still widely prescribed, are also being re-evaluated because they do not benefit everyone[24] as a preventive approach to heart attack and other forms of heart disease, and because of the serious side effects they can cause.[25]

Increasingly, scientists and physicians alike are pointing out that high blood cholesterol by itself is not so much the problem in coronary artery disease as inflammation.[26] They are recognizing that C-reactive protein levels are a clearer predictor of cardiac events[27] and that chronic inflammation is the equally, if not more, serious issue in heart disease.[28]

One of the main reasons for this shift in emphasis is because cholesterol in the body poses a risk only when it oxidizes, a process similar to rust. Oxidation of cholesterol is linked with inflammation, which scientists have now shown is increased by the low-fat, carbohydrate-rich diets once recommended to prevent heart disease.[29,30]

Interestingly, even inflammation may be a secondary risk factor. As noted in Chapter 2, Dr. Cowan, who has researched heart disease and its causes for many years, has found that the primary cause of heart disease, including heart attack and stroke, is diminished functioning of the parasympathetic nervous system.[31]

Dr. Cowan is not alone in his views. In fact, the primary role that diminished parasympathetic nervous system functioning plays in the onset of heart disease has been discussed in prestigious mainstream medical journals, including *Circulation* and the *Journal of Cardiology.*

In a 2008 *Circulation* article,[32] the authors wrote, "Abundant evidence links sympathetic nervous system activation to outcomes of patients with heart failure (HF). In contrast, parasympathetic activation has complex cardiovascular effects that are only beginning to be recognized."

In summarizing their medical findings related to diminished parasympathetic activity and heart failure, the authors concluded, "Autonomic regulation of the heart has an important influence on the progression of HF. Although elevated sympathetic activity is associated with an adverse prognosis, a high level of parasympathetic activation confers cardio protection by several potential mechanisms. These parasympathetic actions on the heart are mediated not only by the direct consequences of cardiac muscarinic receptor stimulation, but also by a multitude of indirect mechanisms.."

Muscarinic receptors help produce parasympathetic effects, such as a slowed heart rate and increased activity of smooth muscle tissue lining the arteries.

Research from 2012, published in the *Journal of Cardiology*,[33] said, "In heart failure, it has been recognized that the sympathetic nervous system (SNS) is activated and the imbalance of the activity of the SNS and vagal activity interaction occurs. The abnormal activation of the SNS leads to further worsening of heart failure...In conclusion, we must recognize that heart failure is a complex syndrome with an autonomic nervous system dysfunction, and that the autonomic imbalance with the activation of the SNS and the reduction of vagal activity should be treated."

In his article "What Causes Heart Attacks,"[34] Dr. Cowan outlined the sequence of events that leads to a heart attack:

"First comes a decrease in the tonic, healing activity of the parasympathetic nervous system—in the vast majority of cases the pathology for heart attack will not proceed unless this condition is met...Then comes an increase in the sympathetic nervous system activity, usually a physical or emotional stressor. This increase in sympathetic activity cannot be balanced because of chronic parasympathetic suppression.

"The result is an uncontrolled increase of adrenaline, which directs the myocardial cells to break down glucose using aerobic glycolysis...As a result of the sympathetic increase and resulting glycolysis, a dramatic increase in lactic acid production occurs in the myocardial cells; this happens in virtually one hundred percent of heart attacks, with no coronary artery mechanism required...

"As a result of the increase in lactic acid in the myocardial cells, a localized acidosis occurs. This acidosis prevents calcium from entering the cells, making the cells less able to contract. This inability to contract causes localized edema (swelling), dysfunction of the walls of the heart (hypokinesis, which is the hallmark of ischemic disease as seen on stress echoes and nuclear thallium stress tests) and eventually necrosis of the tissue—in other words, a heart attack...

"The localized tissue edema also alters the hemodynamics of the arteries embedded in that section of the heart, resulting in shear pressure, which causes the unstable plaques to rupture, further block the artery, and worsen the hemodynamics in that area of the heart.

"Please note that this explanation alone explains why plaques rupture, what their role in the heart attack process is, and why they should indeed be addressed. Notice also that this explanation accounts for all the observable phenomena associated with heart disease and is substantiated by years of research. It could not be clearer as to the true origin of this epidemic of heart disease."

Dr. Cowan concludes his article by stating:

"If heart disease is fundamentally caused by a deficiency in the parasympathetic nervous system, then the solution is obviously to nurture and protect that system, which is the same as saying we should nurture and protect ourselves. Nourishing our parasympathetic nervous system is basically the same as dismantling a way of life for which humans are ill-suited."

Based on all of the above, and given how effectively and predictably NuCalm creates a state of parasympathetic nervous system dominance, you can understand why regular NuCalm use can be a very important step in reducing the risk of heart disease and improving overall cardiovascular function.

As an example of just how powerful regular use of NuCalm can be with regard to heart disease, consider the case of one of Dr. Holloway's patients.

"This was maybe the most extraordinary case I've had with NuCalm," Dr. Holloway said. "It involved a man who came to me after suffering a very severe heart attack. He had been treated at one of the big heart hospitals in Houston and when you looked at the SPECT scan (3-D nuclear imaging) of his heart, you could see that his heart had sustained significant muscle damage. This guy was very wealthy. He was an extremely Type A personality, and he had a lot of anger. He was what I call a 'rager,' and treated people very poorly. Quite frankly, I didn't much want to work with him. Any time I'm judging like that, though, I try to reign back on myself and know that it's not about me and not necessarily about him, but he was not a very pleasant guy when he came to see me.

"When I first met with him, I told him, 'I've got something I think might help but I really don't want to bring it out and show it to you because I don't think that you would have the capacity to do it.' He raised up to aggressively lean forward in his chair and said, 'There's nothing I can't do if I decide to do it.' I said, 'OK, we can find out.' So over a period of about four months, I gave him regular NuCalm sessions, along with a program of orthomolecular nutrition and some heart rate variability exercises.

"Like many people who are ragers, this man, deep down, was really pretty scared to death when I began working with him. But during those four months or so, the most extraordinary transformation began to occur in him. This was a man who didn't know a thing in the world about love. He just knew how to con and manipulate people to get what he wanted. He was afraid to act any differently. But all of that changed, the more that he did NuCalm. For the first time in his adult life, he found that he was able to open himself up to being kinder and more trusting, and not only focused on himself. As I say, he experienced an extraordinary transformation in his personality.

"And then, about six months after he first came to me, he went in to have another heart scan. Both he and his doctors were astonished to discover that there was no longer any evidence of damage in his heart muscle. That was very much related to the personality transformation that he had, which was entirely due to how his NuCalm sessions took him out of the perpetual state of fight-or-flight mode he had operated under. After that, he was a completely changed man in terms of how he conducted himself in his personal and professional life."

Sleep Disorders

Lack of quality sleep is a big problem for many people today. In fact, one-third of American adults have brief bouts of insomnia, some 20 percent have disturbed sleep for up to three months at a time and 10 percent have chronic insomnia disorder.[35] Too many people can't fall asleep, wake up in the middle of the night, or toss and turn, only to greet the morning feeling exhausted.

The importance of a good night's sleep cannot be overemphasized. Lack of sleep has been implicated in a wide range of health problems, including lowered immunity and a greater susceptibility to infections, increased stress and muscle tension, increased weight gain, impaired brain function, and increased risk of heart disease and certain types of cancer. It increases the risk of developing Type 2 diabetes, hormonal imbalances and high blood pressure. Lack of sleep also leads to a diminished ability to solve problems, decreased creativity, reduced productivity and poor job performance.[36,37]

A primary cause of sleep disorders is overstimulation of the sympathetic nervous system. Given NuCalm's proven ability to correct this problem, it should not be surprising that a commonly reported benefit is deep, restful sleep. Most users notice this improvement after only a few sessions of NuCalm. It's no surprise either, as both the NuCalm supplement formula and calming cream include the amino acid GABA, the most important inhibitory neurotransmitter in the brain, which helps prevent over-firing of nerve cells. Through its metabolic processes, the brain uses GABA to create tranquility and calmness, supporting a relaxed state of mind and thus promoting healthy sleep.

The sleep-promoting benefits that GABA provides are increased significantly when combined with CES and NuCalm's proprietary neuroacoustics. The following case histories illustrate how powerfully this unique combination of components can help achieve restorative sleep.

The first case involves a family from Arizona attending the cancer health camp we discussed earlier in this chapter. Not only did this family have a little girl who was undergoing cancer treatments, but her sibling had severe ADHD. The mother told one of the camp counselors just how challenging it was at nighttime for her and her family to get their much-needed sleep. She explained that the ADHD child would run around and refuse to lie quietly and stay in his bed. The counselor told her about NuCalm and provided the system to her.

That night she took the NuCalm headset and placed it on her overactive child's head, then went in the other room for only a few minutes. When she came back, the child was sound asleep and in fact did not move until she physically woke him the next morning. She was adamant that this had never happened before, and told the counselor that she and her entire family all had the most restful night's sleep she could remember.

In the second case, a 36-year-old recovery patient of Dr. Holloway accepted a promotion to a supervisory position at the warehouse where he worked. The patient was excited to make progress toward a management job, but the shift he now supervised was at night. His circadian rhythms were thrown off by several hours and he had great difficulty getting sufficient sleep. In order to help, Dr. Holloway combined NuCalm with instructions for lowering ambient lighting and other sleep preparation methods. The patient was able to adjust to the new routine and rest well, despite the demands of his new work cycle.

Jet Lag

Jet lag is another form of sleep disorder. Known as *circadian dysrhythmia* or *desynchronosis*, it refers to an imbalance of our normal 24-hour circadian rhythm. If you've ever experienced jet lag, you know how it can disrupt your sleep and make you feel off your game. Here is a closer look at its causes.

Circadian rhythms are influenced by various hormones, released at specific times throughout the day and night in the body's 24-hour cycle. The main biological clock that regulates these rhythms is found within the nucleus of the hypothalamus, next to the midbrain region. Among its functions, the hypothalamus ensures that each hormone is produced and secreted at the proper time. These hormones control alertness, sleepiness, mood, pain threshold, energy levels, body temperature and sex drive.

For example, if you normally go to bed at 11 p.m., your hypothalamus signals a release of melatonin at around 10:30 p.m. and causes your body temperature to drop in preparation for sleep. At around 4 a.m., your body reaches its lowest temperature. Then, to prepare you for waking, your hypothalamus signals a release of cortisol around 6 a.m., followed by adrenaline a short time later.

When you travel by plane and fly faster than the rotation of the earth, particularly when you fly against the direction of the earth's rotation, your body is forced into a transient state. You experience mental and cellular chaos as your body rhythms reluctantly break their normal daily patterns, struggle to adapt, and shift into a new time zone.

This shift causes a major disruption in the synchronization of the body rhythms that keep your heart pumping to one rhythm, while your lungs inhale and exhale to another. All the normal signals within your body are affected, including those that release enzymes and stomach acids in anticipation of eating, that put your body to sleep at night, that wake you in the morning, and that control the timing of every other function of your body, right down to the cellular level.

This event of desynchronization or jet lag is the period during which your body recalibrates its biorhythms, attempting to adjust to a different time and place.

Here are the typical periods necessary to complete this re-calibration after a two-hour time zone change flying east:

- Performance (psychomotor)—3 days
- Reaction time (vigilance)—1 to 2 days
- Heart rate—2 days
- Corticosteroids (urinary)—4 days
- Noradrenaline (urinary)—1 day
- Adrenaline (urinary)—2 days
- Bowel movements—3 days
- Body temperature—3 days
- Sleep pattern—1 day.

People who fly frequently, especially experienced pilots who are subjected to the additional stresses that accompany their profession, report that using NuCalm before, during and/or after flying does an exceptional job of alleviating the stress of jet lag. It quickly restores order to their body rhythms and timing mechanisms. Research shows that a 45-minute NuCalm session restores homeostasis to the entire autonomic nervous system[38] while rapidly resetting the body's biological clocks.

What follows are the observations of a very experienced pilot over a four-week period, after he first was introduced to and began using NuCalm. At the time of this writing, the 44-year-old had been a professional pilot for 21 years and had logged more than 14,000 hours of flight time. Currently, he is a private jet pilot and flies twice a month from Los Angeles to Sydney, Australia, to Tel Aviv, Israel, and back to Los Angeles. He also pilots planes domestically several times per week.

Initial experience: "My colleague (co-pilot) tried NuCalm first before our departure. He used it for 14 minutes before we had to depart. He did not take the NuCalm supplements, only using the eye mask with the CES unit and the music headset. I had to wake him up, and his first reaction was to exclaim, 'Wow!'

"While he was using the unit, I took three supplement tablets and chewed them for about a minute. Once we lifted off and reached cruising level, about 40 minutes after I chewed the tablets, I used NuCalm for 36 minutes. Throughout the rest of the five-hour flight, I was alert and felt rested, even though I had minimum sleep the previous two nights. I am used to sleeping after sunset, as my body has accustomed itself to wake during daylight hours and sleep during night hours. Normally, I would struggle extremely hard to stay awake during this type of flight. I was quite impressed with my first NuCalm experience and resolved to keep using NuCalm."

Second experience: "I used NuCalm last night for about 45 minutes. At first, I could not relax. After that, my mind seemed to be drifting fast and I realized I was daydreaming. I am writing this at 5 a.m. after just waking up, feeling the most rested that I can ever remember being. I actually slept through the night for the first time in over ten years. I do believe this will be a game changer for the type of flying my colleagues and I do."

Observations, Week 2: "I am on the second bottle of NuCalm supplements now. Since I began using NuCalm, I continue to receive positive feedback from my colleagues who are now also using NuCalm. Here is a sampling of their comments to me. 'I'm getting the best sleep I've ever had during the nights when I use it before bed.' 'Within 20 minutes I can go from full speed to being completely relaxed.' 'Wow! That was the best 15 minutes ever!'" (Right after this pilot used NuCalm for that length of time.)

Observations, Week 4: "I gave a NuCalm unit to a UPS crew to use for two weeks. They used it for flights originating out of Anchorage, Alaska, to China and report that they 'absolutely love it!' My crew and I are using it on the current flight that I am on now. The flight attendant demands that we keep the (NuCalm) unit on board. I have another crew within our company who will also begin using it on their international flights.

"Using NuCalm has made me realize two things: How good it feels to not be stressed and how important a good night's sleep is. I feel ten years younger and am doing everything better."

NuCalm as an Aid for Other Conditions

NuCalm is not a medical device designed to diagnose, treat or cure disease. However, as you have learned from the case histories and testimonials we've shared thus far in this chapter, using it regularly can help to improve health outcomes. This is because NuCalm turns off the body's stress response. It upregulates the parasympathetic nervous system, thus reversing sympathetic nervous system dominance. Indirectly, these NuCalm benefits help bolster the body's own healing response.

"Healing is more difficult when we are chronically stressed and in a state of sympathetic nervous system dominance," Dr. Holloway said. "In the sympathetically dominant state, your body is flooded with stress chemicals which, if this process becomes chronic, can compromise immune function and negatively impact the body's other healing mechanisms, as well.

"Ongoing sympathetic dominance due to stress is a significant causative and exacerbating factor in many of the chronic diseases that we see today, including chronic fatigue, autoimmune conditions such as lupus and multiple sclerosis, as well as a wide range of other conditions, including many cases of gastrointestinal disorders, and even skin conditions such as psoriasis.

"For example, one of my patients was an older woman who came to me suffering from a horrible outbreak of psoriasis. She was also married to a man who treated her very badly and really was verbally abusive. She did not come to me to treat her psoriasis, but to find help in dealing with all of the stress she was under because of her marriage.

"I gave her three NuCalm sessions over a period of ten days. Her stress levels were greatly reduced as a result, but what was most surprising to me was that her psoriasis cleared up as well. It usually takes many weeks for psoriasis as bad as hers to clear up, and usually drastic dietary changes and other measures must be used. I didn't do any of that for this woman because I was simply helping her de-stress. Yet her use of NuCalm still resulted in significantly improved skin health in that short time."

Another example of NuCalm's health-enhancing benefits is in this testimonial from the wife of a Connecticut man who experienced severe, unhealthy weight loss due to complications caused by Lyme disease. She wrote, "My husband has been losing weight for eight months, dropping 50 pounds to only weigh 120 pounds on a 5-foot-8 frame. Believing it was a manifestation of Lyme disease attacking his gastrointestinal system, we tried several alternative treatments, trying to avoid antibiotics. His weight loss all started with violent vomiting and he was often in pain after eating. It became a pattern to vomit whenever his stomach hurt. He literally became afraid to eat and quite drastically reduced his food intake, and that's when his weight loss spiral began.

"As a last resort attempt to find a solution and stop the weight loss, we consulted with Cheryl Larson, a local health practitioner. She sensed that my husband had a tightly constricted esophageal area near his chest, and recommended that he use the NuCalm technology to help with his stress. This constriction has now released and relaxed as a result of his NuCalm sessions. After only using the NuCalm therapy eight times, he is back to eating normally without any pain and no more vomiting! We expect to continue using this technology as he endeavors to regain lean muscle mass."

A practitioner of craniosacral therapy, with extensive training in CST and other healing modalities, Larson offered her own impressions of NuCalm, saying, "My experience with NuCalm began in June of 2015, when a colleague shared this amazing technology with me. She asked me to experience NuCalm and give her my feedback on it. With a bit of hesitation, I thought, 'Nothing is as calming as an advanced craniosacral therapy session, but I'll give it a try.' Well, I quickly learned that NuCalm was significantly more relaxing. The four components of NuCalm seemed too elementary to provide such an impactful experience.

"When I NuCalmed, my thoughts and absolute sense of comfort were effortless. My curious mind was hard at work observing my brain, which felt like it was being rewired without the stressful tension that normally accumulates and leaves me tired, scattered and not centered or grounded. It was as if I was receiving a CST session: very relaxing, very natural and serene. I recognized some deeper inhalations as well as physical releases of tensions I had been holding onto with a tight grip. I slipped into a deep alpha-theta state without hesitation or effort. After 57 minutes, which somehow seemed like 15 minutes, I suddenly awoke feeling like I was awake and ready to go. I was in awe, and wanted to know more.

"I work with the brain and the central nervous system as a therapist using a technique called craniosacral therapy, which I have been effectively using for 25 years. I possess a great deal of expertise in the craniosacral system, somato-emotional release, neurotransmitters and the neuroscience of the brain. The ability to palpate or feel the internal landscape of a person's brain and spinal cord is not to be taken lightly. This skill and privilege comes with the discipline and intention to pay close attention to what I can feel with my hands using a light touch.

"I started to explore NuCalm on my patients while I engaged them in CST sessions. Before I set up NuCalm, I will routinely observe my patients' SQAR: symmetry, quality, amplitude and rate of the craniosacral rhythm; as well as neurotransmitter responses such as dopamine, acetylcholine, GABA and serotonin. Then I administer NuCalm.

"After three minutes on NuCalm, I place my hands under the patient's cranial base and sacral base and listen for the CST rhythm. I can feel a complete still point. This is incredible, because achieving a still point typically takes a full CST session or more! A still point is a pause in the cerebral spinal fluid flow, allowing the nervous system to relax. As I check into the brain of a patient on NuCalm, it's as if the neurotransmitters are building a matrix of connections together. This is a powerful thing when it comes to the health of a brain. We all need this to help us heal.

"On a personal note, I've experienced my own trials, tribulations and traumas, such as a head injury. Using NuCalm has given me a whole new perspective and has facilitated my own healing. Having remnants of a severe concussion is frustrating to say the least. I have experienced wonderful results over the years from CST and other modalities of treatment, but the day I experienced NuCalm was a day of amazement and excited joy to feel my brain healing. With NuCalm, I routinely experience the sensations of repair and renewal, and can feel clarity and calm coming together.

"I see this NuCalm technology as an adjunct to any professional practice. Health and wellness will be the greatest result. I extend a big thank you to Dr. Blake Holloway. What he has developed with NuCalm is innovation at its finest. Imagine the possibilities that NuCalm has. The world is a better place when the human race calms down."

As you learned earlier in the section on dental procedures, the use of NuCalm also appears to enhance the healing of wounds. Wound healing is the body's natural restorative response to tissue injury.

This healing process itself is a complex system of cascading events at the cellular level that result in a temporary and necessary localized inflammation in order to repair the wound site. Impediments to any of these cellular functions during the healing process can delay healing and compromise the outcome.

A quick on-line search yields myriad scientific articles about stress and its profoundly negative impact on the body's response systems, down to the cellular level. Chronic stress, with its ongoing production of stress hormones, impairs the healing process and slows it down. Research has found that sustained, elevated levels of the stress hormone cortisol not only decrease the inflammatory response associated with wound healing, but also suppress immune function, thus increasing the risk of infection within the wound site.[39]

Given what you now know about NuCalm's proven ability to resolve stress, you can understand how and why NuCalm may have significant potential as an aid to wound healing beyond that already demonstrated with NuCalm's use during intense dental surgical procedures.

In the future, more studies related to NuCalm and its potential health-related benefits will continue with cancer patients, and likely expand into other patient groups where one of the disease components is stress. What remains clear is that because of how it arrests and reverses chronic stress, NuCalm can provide adjunctive support to interrupt several of the steps on the pathway to illness, as well as bolster the healing response of people suffering from disease.

We end this chapter with comments by Tarman Aziz, M.D., a former professor of neuroscience, now consulting in Michigan on stress and the immune system. Dr. Aziz has used NuCalm extensively and summarized its potential health benefits as follows:

"The ability of NuCalm to reduce sympathetic discharge, and its impact on the autonomic nervous system, is clearly a freestanding and noteworthy contribution to society and our high-paced, stress-filled lives. We know that every organ system in the human body is disturbed when sympathetic tone predominates excessively and chronically. It therefore seems logical to run with the research on NuCalm already in place and start measuring the possible reduction, with long-term NuCalm use, of predictable organ and systemic dysfunction.

"I believe, with using NuCalm, that three weeks of reduced sympathetic discharge should make significant improvements to the body's white blood cell population's ability to process foreign invaders in the lymph nodes. We all have experienced the sore throat and generally run-down feeling one can get after a few nights of bad sleep. The sympathetic discharge associated with sleep deprivation and long working hours under stress allows opportunistic viruses and bacteria to colonize and challenge our immune system.

"When confronted with chronic inflammatory conditions, cancer, bacterial-viral infections, and other assaults to the body's homeostasis, it becomes critical to optimize the immune system. I can imagine a myriad of uses for NuCalm to demonstrate the immune-boosting role of shifting to a parasympathetic-dominated tone."

We agree.

Chapter 6

PERFORMANCE AND CREATIVITY

Chronic stress can and does negatively influence all areas of your life: physical, emotional and beyond. The problems it creates inevitably improve when you are able to manage stress successfully. Meeting your daily life challenges with confidence and enthusiasm becomes easier. This is precisely what regular users of NuCalm report.

In this chapter, we discuss some of the other aspects of life, in addition to the health benefits, that NuCalm may enhance. Specifically, we will examine how NuCalm can improve your personal and professional performance, your physical and athletic ability, your creativity, and your ability to solve life's daily challenges and problems.

Personal and Professional Performance

Many high-powered executives and people of influence today use the NuCalm technology to improve their personal and professional performance, manage stress and quickly capture many of the same benefits that usually are achieved only by long-term meditators.

When it comes to personal and professional performance, no one is more renowned than global icon, motivational pioneer and philanthropist Anthony Robbins. He became a regular user of NuCalm as soon as Dr. Galitzer first introduced him to it in May 2015.

In October 2015, *Business Insider* profiled Robbins with an article entitled, "Tony Robbins Explains How He Sustains a Massive Amount of Energy with No Stimulants and Little Sleep." Robbins was described as "a fan of the NuCalm system," continuing "...that in the previous day's media circuit, he had just a half-hour window of free time, and he chose to use NuCalm for 20 of those minutes and felt rejuvenated." The author of the profile concluded the section on

Robbins' use of NuCalm by writing, "The main takeaway: If you can find a way to enter a deep meditative state for 20 minutes, your body may feel refreshed and rid of debilitating stress."

One of the primary factors that separates poor performers from peak performers is how each group deals with the stress and anxiety that can arise in those moments of truth, when what they seek to achieve is within their grasp. While peak performers may experience stress and anxiety at such times, they simply acknowledge that fact and do not let such emotions stand in their way. They have developed and honed success traits that enable them to produce the results they want.

By contrast, all too many people allow stress and anxiety to cripple them, forestalling the success they hope for, even when they possess all the skills they need to achieve it. One such example was a client of Dr. Holloway.

"This man came to me after failing to pass his bar exam here in Texas," Dr. Holloway said. "Not only did he fail the exam, he was unable to even finish taking it, that's how great his anxiety was. He suffered from one of the most severe cases of 'test anxiety' I'd ever witnessed. Yet all through college and law school, he had been a 4.0 student and had graduated at the top of his class. His instructors considered him a shoo-in to pass the bar, and he certainly possessed all the knowledge he needed to do so. But the very thought of taking the exam itself caused him great anxiety. The first time he sat for the bar, his anxiety was so great that, within the first 45 minutes, his shirt was soaked through with sweat and he got up and fled the room.

"To help him prepare to sit for the bar a second time, I introduced him to NuCalm and gave him NuCalm sessions twice a day. I also had his wife give him NuCalm sessions during test breaks during the exam, which is administered over three days.

"As a result, this time he was able to sit for the bar successfully, and when he received his results, he found out that he'd aced it. And the Texas bar exam is one of the toughest of any state because of all the gas and oil laws we have in Texas, as well as complex family law, and so forth.

"The difference that NuCalm made for this man was remarkable. Before NuCalm, he was a basket case of nerves; after NuCalm, he was calmly able to call upon all of the knowledge he had gained during his education and pass the bar with flying colors."

Though the above case is admittedly extreme, NuCalm helped this man achieve results like those reported by other business professionals who use NuCalm to help them master what Tony Robbins calls "the winning edge." This is true, as well, for Jim Poole, the CEO of Solace Lifesciences, and is why he is so committed to helping Dr. Holloway bring the benefits of NuCalm to the world.

We conclude this section with a testimonial from Jim Poole that explains the significant difference NuCalm has made, and continues to make, in both his professional and personal life.

"Before NuCalm, my business partner Chris Gross and I were running Focused Evolution, a strategy consulting firm with an expertise in mergers and acquisitions, due diligence, and growth strategies for venture capital and private equity firms. Under my leadership, Focused Evolution grew into a multimillion-dollar consulting firm serving a global client portfolio of 49 companies in several industries, including health care, biotechnology, market research, dental and IT. We successfully launched global products and businesses, managed growth strategies, and effectively optimized business operations for both large and small organizations across the business lifecycle.

"While the rewards were great and we enjoyed the challenges that came our way, the amount of stress we faced on a regular basis running companies around the world was immense. On top of that, my job entailed too much air travel across multiple time zones on a regular basis, leaving me exhausted. My body and mind could only do so much before I would feel myself breaking down, losing my patience, making important business decisions clouded by emotion, and simply not operating at my best. I never felt grounded, even if I was home for a few days.

"The stress also affected my personal life. I found it difficult to shut off my brain and compartmentalize my business challenges when I was home so I could focus on my beautiful family. I tried to maintain a healthy diet and exercise, but was not sleeping well and was drinking too much alcohol, probably to try and escape from my stress and overactive mind. My relationships at home suffered, and how could they not? It's funny, you don't really notice, or pay attention to, all of this, until stress no longer consumes you and you can reflect on what used to be 'normal.'

"In the end, though, my journey and sacrifice at Focused Evolution may have been worth it, as it led me to meet Dr. Blake Holloway. In June 2009, Blake came to Focused Evolution wanting our help. That, in and of itself, was not unique as Focused Evolution had a reputation for helping small businesses grow, and many small businesses asked for our help. What I found unique was Blake's intellectual horsepower, compassion and humility.

"I immediately liked Blake as a person and then he said, 'I have developed a technology that can quickly, effectively and safely relax the mind and body within minutes without drugs or side effects.' I had never heard such a statement and my curiosity was piqued enough to engage our firm in three months of intense due diligence. In October, Chris and I flew to Texas to try this technology for ourselves because it sounded too good to be true.

"My first NuCalm experience was profound. I had no idea how it did what it did, but my jet lag was immediately erased, my body felt a sense of relaxation I didn't recognize, yet my mind was clear

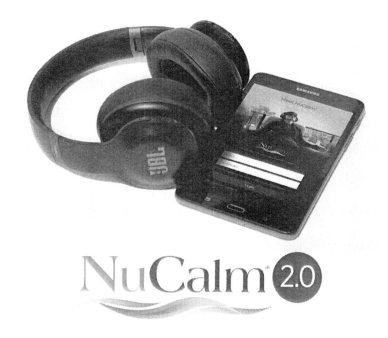

and inspired. After a couple weeks of using NuCalm, I could feel a noticeable shift in my life, both professionally and personally. Things that used to bother me were no longer bothering me. Interpersonal conflict was easy to resolve without emotional entanglement. My sleep was drastically improved, thus my positive energy every day was greater. My eating choices on the road were better and I was drinking less. And most importantly, when I was home, I was home...focused on my wife and three children, totally engaged, laughing, playing, listening and loving!

"Life is fast, and every year it seems to go by faster. Our pace as a society is accelerating yet untenable, but we're not slowing down. This technology slowed me down, on the inside, which actually facilitated greater efficiencies, clarity and patience on the outside. Within just four weeks, we intrinsically knew we had to stop everything else and focus on bringing this technology to the world. It was a big decision... to shut down a global consulting firm that had consumed our lives for years, and focus our attention on changing the world through a technology the world had never seen.

"As you might imagine, the challenges of bringing to market a new technology during the precarious and fearful economic times of 2009, with limited resources and nothing but debt, were profound. If I feared failure, I wouldn't have signed on as president and CEO of the company. To be honest, my career running companies required tremendous locus of control, vision, organization, determination, communication and perseverance.

"For the first time in my career, I don't feel like I control the destiny of Solace Lifesciences, I simply am conducting the orchestration of bringing to the world a technology humanity desperately needs, even if it doesn't know it. I use NuCalm every day when I travel and a couple of times per week when I'm home. I am not the same person I used to be. I am balanced, healthy, present in the moment without judgment, focused, happy and resilient. I love my family, I love my business team, I love NuCalm and I love seeing the profound impact NuCalm is having on the world! I'm really excited about the NuCalm 2.0 app, our first move from a premium Class III medical device to versions that are more accessible to more people. I view NuCalm as a gift from Dr. Holloway and it is my obligation to bring this amazing technology to the world."

Physical and Athletic Performance

When stress is properly managed, physical performance improves. For this reason, NuCalm is becoming increasingly popular among professional athletes who need to stay mentally sharp, and be able to achieve and maintain peak physical performance. These world-class athletes use NuCalm because it significantly enhances their ability to manage stress, which improves their muscle recovery, healing and quality of sleep.

At the time of this writing, NuCalm is being used by athletes on 18 professional sports teams in the United States. Professional golfers, boxers, tennis players and MMA fighters also are using NuCalm.

As an example of the benefits NuCalm can provide athletes, consider this case history from competitive swimmer Sarah Bofinger, who is also a personal fitness and swimming coach, and owner of Superstar Fitness LLC.

"I am a competitive swimmer and am training to qualify for the 2020 Olympics," Bofinger said. "I was born with hip dysplasia and have had seven total hip surgeries. Recently, I have had a lot of success using NuCalm to aid in my recovery and mental focus.

"I first discovered NuCalm from my dentist in April 2015. She told me how athletes were using it for recovery, sleep quality and focus. I was immediately interested and wanted to learn more. She put me in contact with the company that makes NuCalm so I could have my questions answered.

"In June 2015, I spoke with Kenton Cowdry, director of client services at Solace Lifesciences Inc. Kenton was very informative about NuCalm and went into depth about how it works. He then connected me with David Poole, who works more with athletes, so David could go into more details on how NuCalm could help me personally. I was amazed by everything David was telling me. At that moment, I was convinced NuCalm was the recovery tool I needed.

"On July 17, 2015, I tried NuCalm for the first time. I felt extremely relaxed and focused. I had a swim meet the next day and wanted to see how I would feel. The morning of the race, I felt very rested and prepared to swim. I got to the race and felt more focused than I had for any other race I can remember. Usually I get really nervous before I swim and can feel my body tense up. NuCalm made me feel so focused and relaxed, I never even thought about being nervous. I swam well and knew if I continued using NuCalm I would feel even better.

"The month of July, I had a race every weekend. After a race, I usually take an ice bath to relieve my inflammation, which can be severe. After just three NuCalm experiences, I did not have to take an ice bath at all! I recovered so much faster than I ever have before.

"I currently use NuCalm just once a week, and twice if I have a race or an intense training week. In August, I competed in my fourth iron girl triathlon and I placed second overall in the swim portion. This was my first triathlon that I did not need to take an ice bath before or after. In addition to minimizing my pain, I cut two minutes off my run and overall time, and felt great the next day. I have only been using NuCalm for two months and I already see amazing benefits. I'm not in as much pain and I don't have to do as much acupuncture, massage and chiropractic treatment. I'm so excited about my future with NuCalm."

After Bofinger wrote the testimonial above, she sent Jim Poole the following email updates:

October 8, 2015: "I have my first USA Swimming race tomorrow. I have decided to use NuCalm just four hours before the race. It really helps with my mental focus for the race. I'll let you know my results."

October 10, 2015: "I rocked my race yesterday! My time in the 1000 freestyle was 11:43:52! I placed first in my heat, and am waiting for overall results. I'm not far from my first cut in that event! I definitely love using NuCalm on race day! I'm always so nervous, but NuCalm gets me right into being race-ready. I don't think. I just swim!"

As mentioned, the Chicago Blackhawks are one of the professional sports teams that use NuCalm to improve performance. The Blackhawks' trainers and players alike credit NuCalm with helping them win the Stanley Cup in 2013 and 2015.

During a two-month period in the 2015 regular NHL hockey season, Solace Lifesciences collected data on several Blackhawks players who use NuCalm. Testing measures were the same as those used to collect data on NuCalm's benefits for stage 4 cancer patients (see Chapter 5). The data sets from one of the Blackhawks players are reflected in the adjacent illustration. This player now has been using NuCalm regularly for more than two years.

In the results from this data, the LF/HF ratio quantifies the balance between the sympathetic nervous system (LF) and the para-sympathetic nervous system (HF) in each subject. As mentioned in Chapter 4, sympatho-vagal balance is critical for professional athletes. They need high cortisol-adrenaline sympathetic function to compete at extreme levels. However, they also need effective parasympathetic function for optimal muscle recovery, healing and sleep.

As did the other Blackhawks players in the study, this player consistently registered a significant decrease in the LF/HF ratio across each five-minute segment of NuCalm use and across the duration of each session, indicating optimal healing. As in other studies, the only anomalies occurred when he fell asleep during the session, which elicited spikes in sympathetic nervous system activity so that his body could maintain its normal heartbeat. Typically, when test subjects fall asleep, it lasts for no more than one to four minutes, after which they come up from sleep to experience the deep relaxation associated with theta brain wave function.

The data showed a consistent pattern regarding NuCalm's impact on this player's autonomic nervous system. Within the first five minutes of experiencing NuCalm, he underwent a rapid descent into parasympathetic nervous system dominance, as evidenced by the profound reduction in the total power spectrum and the LF/HF ratio (see chapters 4 and 5).

This player's total power spectrum rapidly decreased, then continued to decrease across each five-minute segment of NuCalm use. This reduction was maintained throughout each of his NuCalm experiences, just as it was among the other Blackhawks players who were tested. In this particular data set, the subject's total power spectrum was reduced by 82 percent within the first five minutes, and by over 96 percent within ten minutes.

Several key observations can be made from this data.

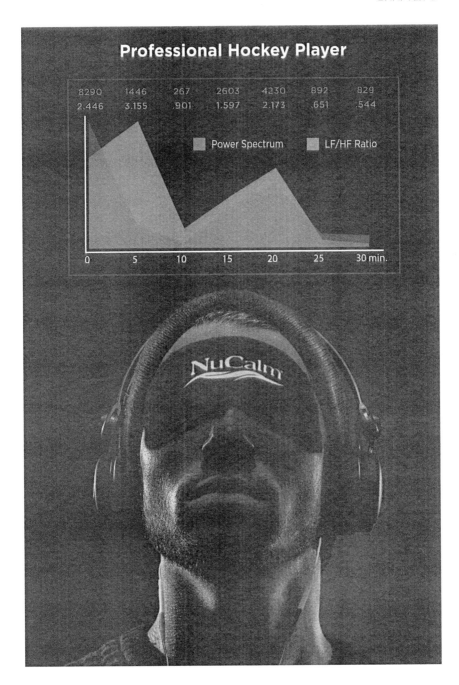

Professional Hockey Player

8290	1446	267	2603	4230	892	829
2.446	3.155	.901	1.597	2.173	.651	.544

■ Power Spectrum   ■ LF/HF Ratio

Blackhawks players tested on NuCalm showed consistent decreases in total power spectrum and LF/HF ratios, marks of parasympathetic dominance. This player's TPS fell 96 percent during his NuCalm session. Spikes result from falling asleep.

First, NuCalm quickly and predictably flips the switch from high cortisol and adrenaline production to deep relaxation. This is important because it allows the body to activate its brain-heart-lung connection, which optimizes diaphragmatic breathing and the flow of oxygen-rich red blood cells, thus maximizing healing and muscle recovery.

Second, the deep relaxation that NuCalm provides throughout the body decreases lactic acid buildup caused by physical activity and, more importantly, reduces inflammation that slows and compromises healing.

Finally, during the course of the regular sports season, and especially during the playoffs, athletes travel across multiple time zones. Such travel can impair both physical and mental performance. NuCalm helps to minimize the effects of such travel by reducing circadian rhythm dysfunction and improving sleep. By restoring autonomic nervous system balance and predictably restoring the body's natural rhythms, NuCalm dramatically assists athletes to perform at their best.

By the end of this two-month study, the Blackhawks players all reported better rates of healing and muscle recovery than those normally experienced prior to using NuCalm. They also observed a marked reduction in symptoms of lactic acid buildup. As one player commented, "I felt loose and relaxed, even after an exhausting workout."

The players also reported significant improvements in the quality of their sleep and experienced little, if any, jet lag. Most importantly, from their perspective, they reported feeling more relaxed during games, despite the pressure that comes with competing at the highest levels of their profession. "My head felt more clear and focused," is how one player summarized his experience on the ice after using NuCalm.

Mike Gapski, the Blackhawks' head trainer introduced in Chapter 1, echoed these sentiments. "You could just tell that these guys were just more relaxed throughout the playoffs, and they would tell me that," Gapski said. "We want our players to play 'intense,' not 'tense,' and NuCalm is a way for them to just relax and effectively deal with frustrations. NuCalm was very beneficial because it clears your head and allows you to start from scratch."

Also introduced in Chapter 1 was Julie Burns, founder and CEO of SportFuel Inc., a Chicago-based integrative sports nutrition practice. Her clients include corporate executives and several Chicago-based professional sports teams.

"NuCalm has proven to be a remarkably reliable tool for helping to modulate cortisol levels and inflammation," Burns said. "NuCalm quickly takes athletes out of their catabolic breakdown mode and shifts them into a healthy build-up mode so they can heal and recover as quickly as possible. When athletes are in a balanced nervous system state, they respond instinctively instead of reacting impulsively, and thereby can perform at their highest level. I count on NuCalm personally, and so do our athletes. They have been using it for over three years and love it."

Among other sports experts and scientists who have observed and studied the effects of NuCalm on professional athletes is Norm Thomas, M.D., D.D.S., Ph.D., O.Path., an Oxford Fellow, and director of neuromuscular research at LVI Global, an advanced dental education institution. Dr. Thomas said, "It is not strength of the musculature that is important in athletic and physical performance, but the relaxation of muscles to produce additional load when required. NuCalm is a significant advancement and an amazing tool for quickly relaxing muscles throughout the entire body."

Creativity and Problem Solving

Improved creativity is another benefit that many users of NuCalm report. "If you talk to long-term NuCalm users, they will frequently share that they are a lot more creative than they were before NuCalm," Dr. Holloway said. "I have a friend who is an author and also, now, a Unitarian minister. Before that, he was a college professor at the doctoral level who had written a major book about Beowulf, as well as other books. He was facing a publication deadline for another book project and found himself stuck with a major case of writer's block.

"Well, one of the things we know about writer's block is that creativity comes when the brain wave level is about 7 Hz, which is associated with high theta frequencies in the brain. I gave this friend a NuCalm session for 90 minutes. As I did so, I monitored his brain wave states in five-minute segments and I could see when he hit that optimal alpha-theta level for creativity. After that session, he went home and he wrote two entire chapters."

Larry Trivieri Jr., co-author of this book, has found NuCalm to be effective for quickly banishing writer's block as well. Trivieri has written or co-written more than 20 health books, has published hundreds of articles and is a children's novelist.

"As a published author for nearly 25 years, I long ago learned to navigate through writer's block, to the point where it rarely affects me today," Trivieri said. "Yet, like most writers, I am still not wholly immune to it, and when it strikes, it can really derail my productivity. A few months after I was first introduced to and began using the NuCalm technology, I was at my computer when suddenly I hit a wall. No matter how I tried, I did not have a clue how to proceed with writing the chapter I was working on. I have a number of tricks, if you will, that I've discovered over the years, that usually allow me to get back into the flow of my writing when writer's block strikes me, but on that day, no matter what I tried, I could not get unstuck.

"I grew increasingly frustrated and, naturally, that only made things worse. Then I realized that I had not given myself a NuCalm session for over a week. As this was the first time I'd experienced writer's block since I'd acquired NuCalm, I was curious to see if it would help me. I turned off my computer and did NuCalm for 20 minutes. By the end of my session, I felt much more energized than I had before. I returned to my computer and immediately started writing again. For the rest of that day's writing session, approximately another four hours, I was in that zone or flow state that all writers relish, and far exceeded my daily writing goal…good-bye writer's block.

"Another benefit that I've gained as a writer using NuCalm is purely physical. When I am absorbed in writing, I oftentimes lose awareness of my physical body. My focus is on what I'm writing, and as a result I can be very much 'in my head' while at my computer.

The end result, when I am done writing for the day, is often a lot of muscular tension, especially in my shoulders, neck and upper back. Typically, I deal with this with a combination of stretching and deep breathing exercises. Now, though, whenever I use NuCalm after I am done writing, soon after I start using it, I can literally feel my muscle tension melting away.

"In addition, thanks to a suggestion Jim Poole made, whenever I experience muscle pain, I rub a little bit of the NuCalm Calming Cream on the sore area. I was surprised the first time I tried this by how much it helped and mentioned it to Jim, who told me that there are GABA receptor sites all over our body, which is why the NuCalm cream provides the relief it does.

"NuCalm hasn't alleviated my muscle tension from writing completely, but it has definitely helped a lot in that respect. Now I make it a point to NuCalm at least three to four times a week, and since I've been doing so, my writing continues to really flow."

Dr. Holloway posits that NuCalm enhances creativity in a number of ways. First, it improves peoples' ability to enter into and regularly access alpha-theta brain wave states, which have long been associated with heightened creativity, inspiration and problem solving. In doing so, NuCalm also improves blood flow to the prefrontal and frontal lobe areas of the brain, which often are referred to as "higher brain" regions because activity there corresponds to higher reasoning, intuition, logic and clear thinking.

Finally, as Dr. Holloway discussed in Chapter 5, NuCalm improves complexity within the autonomic nervous system. "When people use NuCalm they are literally setting the organs of their nervous system up for entirely new potentials," he said. "The more the nervous system and brain are able to operate from higher levels of complexity, the easier it is to solve problems and discover new solutions that previously were not even considered as possibilities.

"When the nervous system loses its ability to operate within higher levels of complexity, which is what occurs when we become habitually stressed, then our ability to effectively solve problems diminishes and we lose time and energy struggling to find solutions. As I like to point out, one of the benefits of using NuCalm is that it improves what is known as the signal-to-noise ratio. Just as computer software needs to be free of noise interference to operate the way it is intended, so too do we need to be free of 'noise' in our nervous system to fully be able to think clearly, solve problems and be creative."

One area where Dr. Holloway would like to see NuCalm introduced is the arena of politics. As the famous quote attributed to Albert Einstein says, "We cannot solve problems using the same kind of thinking we used when we created them." The problems we face in the world today require innovative solutions. Unfortunately, many elected leaders seem incapable of providing them. All too often, they remind us of the quip defining insanity as doing the same thing over and over again, and expecting different results.

One of the reasons world leaders may seem incapable of thinking outside the box for solutions is that they can get locked into fight-or-flight mode. This is evident by the polarized, angry rhetoric that sometimes passes for political discourse. Instead of coming together for a meaningful discussion about the problems facing the world, far too often politicians and world leaders stubbornly hold fast to their own agendas.

"Politics can shut down the brain," Dr. Holloway said. "It doesn't matter if you are on the right or on the left of the political spectrum. Any time you become fixated on one side or the other, your brain's not doing all that it can. We've seen this on brain scans. The brain is in a very stuck place, and it stays stuck because of all of the anger and frustration that so many people experience when they discuss politics. It's a vicious circle. Stuck brains trigger anger and frustration, and anger and frustration keep the brain stuck.

"I don't want furiously angry people running things because, guess what? They don't have enough blood in the front of their brains, where they need it, to truly do their jobs effectively and with reason. You literally cannot solve problems when you are in that state. Instead, you experience emotional resistance to any ideas by which you feel threatened, and that kills creativity and ingenuity.

"I like to remind people that either we can be creative or we can be reactive. The more driven by the sympathetic nervous system that you are, the more reactive and fear-driven you will be. Your ability to solve problems will become virtually nonexistent at that point.

"I often use the example of a hiker in the woods. If he is sympathetically driven, he may see something ahead of him on the trail and jump back in alarm, thinking that it's a snake. But once he calms down and looks again, he discovers it was never a snake, it was just a harmless stick. He was initially unable to perceive this because his brain was operating from its mid and limbic regions, and thus his reasoning and higher faculties of perception were shut off.

"This is the state so many of our leaders today seem to be stuck in. Now imagine what might happen if these same leaders, as well as their politically-fixated and polarized supporters, all could be introduced to NuCalm and start to upregulate their parasympathetic nervous systems. Within a short time, I think we could begin to see a lot more civility in our political discourse, and a lot of new, more creative answers to the problems we and the world face today."

As Solace Lifesciences continues its mission of introducing NuCalm to the world, we, the authors, hope that Dr. Holloway's vision will soon start to become a reality. In the meantime, you do not need to wait for such a paradigm shift to occur. As Mahatma Gandhi wrote in 1913, "If we could change ourselves, the tendencies in the world would also change. As a man changes his own nature, so does the attitude of the world change towards him. ..."

Given the many positive benefits that NuCalm has imparted to the authors, we encourage you to investigate using NuCalm, so that you may experience the dramatic improvements it can make in your ability to manage stress, and to think, function and feel better. We are certain that you will want to make NuCalm a regular part of your overall health and wellness regimen, just as an ever-growing number of health professionals and others like you already are doing.

Thank you for taking the time to read this book. May you and your loved ones regularly experience positive change through rest and relaxation!

Glossary

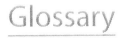

(for the purposes of this book)

Alpha-Theta Crossovers — These occur during brain wave biofeedback, and can be seen on EEGs, when alpha brain waves (8 to 12 Hz) begin crossing with theta brain waves (4 to 8 Hz). These crossovers indicate hypnagogia, the transitional state between wakefulness and sleep, characterized by losing a sense of time and space. This state helps with treatment of stress, anxiety, trauma and addiction.

Amygdala — Parts of the brain responsible for autonomic responses to fear and other emotions, the amygdalae are part of the limbic system and located in each of the medial temporal lobes. When the amygdala is highly stimulated by fear, it purposely shuts off the reasoning area of the brain as it initiates the fight-or-flight response.

Autonomic Nervous System — The autonomic nervous system oversees the health and activity of bodily functions such as heart rate, blood pressure, breathing and digestion, as well as having the fastest and most profound effect on controlling and regulating homeostasis in the body. It is in direct contact with both the central nervous system (brain and spinal cord) and the peripheral nervous system (motor and sensory nerves) and it is comprised of two branches, the sympathetic nervous system and the parasympathetic nervous system. Because it controls the body's ability to react and adapt to stressors and changes, it has great importance to health. Humans need balance in their autonomic nervous system. When it is perpetually out of balance, the body will begin to break down on a cellular level, creating negative consequences.

Binaural Beats — First discovered in mid-1800s, binaural beats involve different neurological pathways than those normally used for hearing. Binaural beats influence brain wave frequencies and can stimulate the production of various hormones and neurochemicals. Typically, the beats are delivered using headphones with one sound frequency played in the left ear and a different frequency played in the right ear. The difference in those frequencies becomes the frequency of the auditory illusion or 'beat' that the brain creates within the superior olivary nuclei. Binaural beats cause the brain's own wave patterns to resonate at that same frequency. If the binaural beat frequency changes, brain wave frequency follows, a phenomenon called frequency-following response or brain wave entrainment. This activates sites in the brain, including the prefrontal and frontal cortices, and can cause the left and right brain hemispheres to harmonize, sometimes referred to as brain hemisphere synchronization. Regular use of binaural beats can bring about a reorganization of the brain itself and its neural pathways, called neuroplasticity.

Brain Wave Entrainment — See binaural beats.

Circadian Dysrhythmia — Also called desynchronosis, circadian dysrhythmia is an imbalance of the body's normal 24-hour circadian rhythm that can be lead to jet lag and other sleep disorders.

Complexity — In the body, complexity is the resilience needed for high-level, robust performance. The more the nervous system and brain are able to operate from higher levels of complexity, the more easily problems are solved and new solutions discovered. When the ability to operate within higher levels of complexity diminishes, which occurs with abnormal stress and sympathetic nervous system dominance, the ability to reason effectively decreases. Any body system losing complexity is going toward entropy or decline, measurable by using heart rate variability and ECG testing. In any disease state, the body is losing complexity.

Cranial Electrotherapy Stimulation (CES) — Through the application of a low, pulsed electric current to specific sites, CES treatments stimulate the brain and brainstem. The current itself is very low and normally is not felt. CES makes brain cell membranes slightly more permeable so that therapeutic substances pass more easily through the membrane into the cell.

Dysautonomia — This is the scientific name for dysfunction of the autonomic nervous system. The body's health, especially the heart and cardiovascular system, is dependent on balanced functioning between the sympathetic and parasympathetic nervous systems. Dysautonomia can be a factor in chronic fatigue syndrome, fibromyalgia, excessively high or low blood pressure, irregular heart rates, irritable bowel syndrome, bladder and urinary problems, sexual function problems and interstitial cystitis. Also see autonomic nervous system.

Evoked Potential — This is the scientific term for the brain's response to specific stimuli, either visual or auditory.

Fight-or-Flight — The body's primal response to a perceived threat, it signals the adrenal glands to increase production of cortisol, adrenaline and other stress hormones, thus allowing quick use of arms and legs to fend off external attacks or get out of harm's way. Blood vessels that supply cells and organs with oxygen and nutrients constrict, so that more blood can flow to tissues in the extremities. Normally, blood is concentrated in the abdominal visceral organs responsible for digestion and absorption of nutrients, for excretion, and for other functions that provide proper cell growth and production of cellular energy. As blood rushes to the extremities, the visceral organs cannot function efficiently, causing all growth-related activities in the body to be limited. Those activities will suffer if this response continues for sustained periods. Unfortunately, thoughts and beliefs also can trigger this response. Although the adrenaline rush caused by an actual physical threat usually does not happen, other aspects of the response still occur and can persist for long periods. This can result in the chronic production of stress hormones and dysautonomia.

Frequency-Following Response — See binaural beats.

GABA — The abbreviation of gamma amino butyric acid, GABA is an inhibitory neurotransmitter that reduces excitability in neurons, promoting a natural state of relaxation. Overstimulated neurons may lead to restlessness, irritability and sleeplessness.

Hertz (Hz) — The international unit of frequency for measuring cyclical waveforms, a hertz equals one cycle per second.

Heart Rate Variability (HRV) — Also known as respiratory sinus arrhythmia, HRV refers to the difference in length of each heartbeat. The more one beat differs from the next, the healthier the heart is. Testing HRV with an electrocardiograph is the simplest and most accurate form of measuring parasympathetic nervous system activity. Heart rate is controlled by brainstem centers including the nucleus ambiguus, which acts with the vagus nerve to increase parasympathetic nervous system signaling to the heart. The heart responds by slowing its beat and exhibiting greater variability. Thus, measuring HRV indicates vagal tone and the level of parasympathetic nervous system activity.

Homeostasis — This is the natural state of stability and balance in the body's functions, down to the cellular level.

HPA axis — An abbreviation for the hypothalamus-pituitary-adrenal axis, this is a key part of the hormonal system. Normally, the HPA axis remains idle, allowing the body to flourish. When the hypothalamus center in the brain perceives an outside threat, it signals the HPA axis to spring into action and initiate the fight-or-flight response. See details under fight-or-flight.

Hypnagogia — See alpha-theta crossovers.

Hypothalamus — This is a small area deep in the brain that acts as the hormone control center and plays a major role is maintaining homeostasis. It is the "H" in HPA axis.

LF/HF Ratio — This is a ratio, found in the results of heart rate variability testing, that quantifiably assesses the balance between the sympathetic nervous system (LF) and parasympathetic nervous system (HF).

Neuroacoustics — This is the science that uses sounds to affect the brain, typically auditory impulses transmitted through headphones to create binaural beats. A different frequency is played in each ear to stimulate the auditory system's frequency following response. The changing of impulse patterns leads to changes in brain wave patterns, or brain wave entrainment, and can produce significant therapeutic results.

Neuroplasticity — This is the scientific term for the brain's capacity to reorganize itself and its neural pathways, which offers a wide range of healthy cognitive and physiological benefits. Within a few daily sessions, treatment with NuCalm can achieve what patients treated within a contemplative neuroscience framework take an average of 90 days to achieve, in terms of positive plastic changes within the brain.

Neurotransmitters — The many types of neurotransmitters are biochemicals used for communication between the brain and the body. Amino acids are their basic building blocks, and they regulate the entire nervous system.

Nuclear Factor Kappa B — A cellular protein involved in DNA structuring, it can act as a genetic inflammatory trigger when a dominant sympathetic nervous system causes overproduction. When sympathetic dominance is chronic, this can lead to a range of unhealthy outcomes, including chronic inflammation and impaired immune function.

Nucleus Ambiguus — This group of motor neurons is the source point of the vagus nerve and, acting with the vagus nerve, increases parasympathetic nervous system signaling to the heart. Because the heart rate is controlled by this and other centers in the brainstem, heart rate variability testing is effective for determining parasympathetic nervous system activity.

Parasympathetic Nervous System — This is the half of the autonomic nervous system devoted to nourishing, healing and rebuilding the body. More active at night, it is engaged in energy recovery, repair, regeneration and relaxation. When actively dominant, it stimulates and enhances immune function, circulation, digestion and overall gastrointestinal function. It improves functioning of the liver, stomach, pancreas and intestines. It also lowers heart rate and blood pressure levels, while increasing production of endorphins, the "feel good" hormones. Achieving and maintaining a healthy parasympathetic state is essential for healing on both the physical and mental-emotional levels. Parasympathetic dominance enables a person to be more relaxed, content and fully present in the moment, as well as able to meet and respond to daily life challenges both calmly and more energetically.

Psychoneuroimmunology (PNI) — PNI often is referred to as mind-body medicine. It continues to identify both the mental, emotional and psychospiritual factors that can predispose people to develop illnesses, such as cancer, and factors that can improve patient outcomes.

Resonant Meditator's Peak — This is another measurement found in heart rate variability testing on NuCalm users. It is found at the 0.1 frequency domain, where brain wave function reaches frequent alpha-theta crossovers and can maintain deep theta. This is the sweet spot for optimizing human biorhythms and is synonymous with 10,000 hours of monastic meditation. When the peak is reached, the body will heal at optimal levels while achieving maximum oxygenated blood flow.

Stress — Any physical, chemical and/or emotional factor causing physical or mental tension that can disrupt the body's equilibrium, thus acting as a primary trigger in the disease process. Stress produces anxiety and inflammation, known to cause chemical and structural changes in the body, including in the circulatory, digestive, endocrine and nervous systems. Chronic stress, with its ongoing production of stress hormones, impairs the healing process.

Superior Olivary Nucleus — The right and left superior olivary nuclei play primary roles in multiple hearing processes and are important to the pathways of the human auditory system. The effects of binaural beats are produced mainly in this area of the brain.

Sympathetic Nervous System — This half of the autonomic nervous system is most active during the day, and is necessary to both energy production and stress-coping mechanisms such as the fight-or-flight response and immune reactions. If dominance of the sympathetic nervous system is maintained indefinitely, which happens with chronic stress, the body stays in fight-or-flight mode, which deprives cells, tissues and organs of needed energy. This can compromise immune function and negatively impact healing mechanisms.

Sympatho-Vagal Balance (LF/HF) — Sympatho-vagal refers to the autonomic nervous system, with *sympatho* being the sympathetic nervous system, and *vagal* referring to the vagus nerve, which is the pathway of the autonomic nervous system and is dominant in the parasympathetic nervous system response. The LF/HF ratio quantifiably assesses the balance between the sympathetic nervous system (LF) and parasympathetic nervous system (HF). Sympatho-vagal balance is imperative for professional athletes, because they need high cortisol-adrenaline sympathetic dominance to compete at extreme levels, as well as parasympathetic nervous system dominance to optimize muscle recovery, healing and sleep quality. Sympatho-vagal balance is important for people battling disease, such as stage 4 cancer, because they must be able to turn off the adrenaline response so that the body can recover and heal. NuCalm restores this balance and regular use can maintain autonomic nervous system health.

Total Power Spectrum — In research concerning the autonomic nervous system using the fast Fourier Transform algorithm, the total power spectrum is found within the frequency-domain results. It is a quantified measure of the autonomic nervous system, both the sympathetic and parasympathetic parts, where the sympathetic tone is the more significant contributor.

Vagus Nerve — This nerve originates in a part of the brainstem called the medulla oblongata and reaches to the colon. It supplies parasympathetic nerve fibers to organs through which it travels, except for the adrenal glands, and is the principal pathway for nerve impulses and signals to and from the parasympathetic nervous system. It regulates the resting state (homeostasis) of most internal organs and the tasks they perform, including heart rate, respiration and gastrointestinal peristalsis. It plays a role in vision, hearing and speech, and controls various skeletal muscles. Vagus nerve activity (vagal tone) and functionality provide a clear indication parasympathetic nervous system activity, especially with regard to heart rate.

Notes

Chapter 1

1. Emma-Jean Weinstein. "Drilling Into Our Fear Of The Dentist — And What To Do About It." *CommonHealth*. WBUR, Boston's NPR News Station, December 20, 2013. http://commonhealth.legacy.wbur.org/2013/12/afraid-of-the-dentist-tips-therapy. [This article quotes Dr. Lisa Heaton, a licensed clinical psychologist at the University of Washington's Dental Fears Research Clinic: https://dental.washington.edu/people/lisa-j-heaton.—Ed.]

2. Richard Sine. "Don't Fear the Dentist." *WebMD*. WebMD LLC, Accessed: August 13, 2016. http://www.webmd.com/oral-health/features/dont-fear-the-dentist. [This archived article quotes Peter Milgrom, doctor of dental surgery, author of *Treating Fearful Dental Patients*, and director of the Dental Fears Research Clinic at the University of Washington: https://dental.washington.edu/people/peter-milgrom. WebMD.com is approved by the URAC, a utilization review accreditation agency.—Ed.]

Chapter 2

1. American Psychological Association, "Stress in America (2015 Survey), Rise in Extreme Stress Accompanies Increase in Stress-Related Symptoms and Poor Health," news release, 2015, APA.org, accessed August 13, 2016, http://apa.org/news/press/releases/stress/2015/snapshot.aspx.

2. Ibid.

3. American Psychological Association, "Stress in America (2015 Survey), Stress Greatly Impacts Adults' Health and Behaviors, Particularly Unhealthy Eating," news release, 2015, APA.org, accessed August 13, 2016, http://apa.org/news/press/releases/stress/2015/snapshot.aspx.

4. Ibid.

5. Ibid.

6. American Psychological Association, "Stress in America (2012 Survey), Impact of Stress," news release, 2012, APA.org, accessed August 13, 2016, https://www.apa.org/news/press/releases/stress/2012/impact-report.pdf.

7. The American Institute of Stress, "Stress Effects," 2011, accessed August 13, 2016, http://www.stress.org/stress-effects.

8. Sheldon Cohen, Denise Janicki-Deverts, and Gregory E. Miller, "Psycho-logical Stress and Disease," *Journal of the American Medical Association* 298, no. 14 (October 10, 2007): 1685-687, accessed August 13, 2016, http:jama.jamanetwork.com/article.aspx?articleid= 209083.

9. "Study of Whitehall Civil Servants Explains How Stress at Work Is Linked to Heart Disease," news release, January 22, 2008, Medical News Today (MNT), accessed August 13, 2016, http://www.medicalnewstoday.com/re-leases/94641.php. [This adapted media release quotes Dr. Tarani Chandola, first author of this Whitehall study, published January 23, 2003 in the Euro-pean Heart Journal.—Ed.]

10. Cancer Facts & Figures 2015. Publication. Atlanta, Georgia: American Cancer Society, 2015. Accessed August 14, 2016. http://www.cancer.org/acs/groups/content/@editorial/documents/document/acspc-044552.pdf.

11. Dariush Mozaffarian et al., "Heart Disease and Stroke Statistics—2015 Update," *Circulation* 131, no. 4 (January 27, 2015): e29-322, Janu-ary 26, 2015, accessed August 13, 2016, doi:http://dx.doi.org/10.1161/CIR.0000000000000152. [*Circulation* is a journal of the American Heart As-sociation aimed at cardiovascular medicine professionals.—Ed.]

12. Ibid., e32.

13. Ibid

14. Ibid., e157.

15. Bruce Lipton, *The Biology of Belief: Unleashing the Power of Conscious-ness, Matter and Miracles*, 10th Anniversary ed. (Carlsbad, California: Hay House, 2008).

16. Harrison Wein, "Stress and Disease: New Perspectives," MedicineN-et, April 6, 2006, accessed August 15, 2016, http://www.medicinenet.com/script/main/art.asp?articlekey=60918. [Article interviews Dr. Esther Stern-berg, who at the time was director of the Integrative Neural Immune Pro-gram at the National Institute of Health's National Institute of Mental Health (NIMH), and whose research demonstrated links between the brain and the immune system.—Ed.]

17. University of Nottingham (UK), University Counselling Office, *What Is the Fight or Flight Response?*, accessed June 15, 2016, https://www.notting-ham.ac.uk/counselling/documents/podacst-fight-or-flight-response.pdf.

18. Sally Guyoncourt, "Chronic Stress Could Lead to Depression and De-mentia, Scientists Warn," *The Independent* (London), January 24, 2016, http://www.independent.co.uk/life-style/health-and-families/health-news/chronic-stress-could-lead-to-depression-and-dementia-scientists-warn-a6831786.html. [Article interviews Dr. Linda Mah, assistant professor

in geriatric psychiatry at the University of Toronto and lead author of the research review, published in full in the journal *Current Opinion in Psychiatry.*—Ed.]

19. Dieter Riemann, "The Hyperarousal Model of Insomnia: A Review of the Concept and Its Evidence," *Sleep Medicine Reviews* 14, no. 1 (February 2010): 19 - 31, http://www.smrv-journal.com/article/S1087-0792(09)00041-0/abstract.

20. Wessel M. A. Van Leeuwen et al., "Sleep Restriction Increases the Risk of Developing Cardiovascular Diseases by Augmenting Proinflammatory Responses through IL-17 and CRP," *PLoS ONE* 4, no. 2 (February 25, 2009), http://dx.doi.org/10.1371/journal.pone.0004589.

21. Alessandro Bartolomucci and Rosario Leopardi, "Stress and Depression: Preclinical Research and Clinical Implications," *PLoS ONE* 4, no. 1 (January 30, 2009), http://dx.doi.org/10.1371/journal.pone.0004265.

22. National Institutes of Health, National Institute of Mental Health, *Any Anxiety Disorder Among Adults*, accessed August 15, 2016, https://www.nimh.nih.gov/health/statistics/prevalence/any-anxiety-disorder-among-adults.shtml.

23. "Understand the Facts: Depression," Anxiety and Depression Association of America, August 2016, https://www.adaa.org/understanding-anxiety/depression.

24. "Facts & Statistics: Did You Know?," Anxiety and Depression Association of America, August 2016, https://www.adaa.org/about-adaa/press-room/facts-statistics.

25. Thomas Insel, "Antidepressants: A Complicated Picture," Director's Blog, National Institute of Mental Health, December 6, 2011, accessed August 17, 2016, http://www.nimh.nih.gov/about/director/2011/antidepressants-a-complicated-picture.shtml.

26. Peter Wehrwein, "Astounding Increase in Antidepressant Use by Americans," *Harvard Health Publications* (blog), Harvard Medical School, October 20, 2011, accessed August 17, 2016, http://www.health.harvard.edu/blog/astounding-increase-in-antidepressant-use-by-americans-201110203624.

27. Tiffany Kary, "Are Antidepressants Addictive?," *Psychology Today,* July 1, 2003, reviewed June 9, 2016, accessed August 17, 2016, https://www.psychologytoday.com/articles/200307/are-antidepressants-addictive.

28. "Understanding Antidepressant Medications: Serious Risks," U.S. Food and Drug Administration, April 13, 2016, accessed August 17, 2016, http://www.fda.gov/forconsumers/consumerupdates/ucm095980.htm.

29. Health Advocate, Inc. and National Women's Health Resource Center, publication from webinar "Health in the Workplace: Meeting the Challenge" (2009), accessed August 17, 2016, http://healthadvocate.com/downloads/webinars/stress-workplace.pdf.

30. Giuseppe Mancia and Guido Grassi, "The Autonomic Nervous System and Hypertension," *Circulation Research* 114, no. 11 (May 23, 2014): 1804-14, accessed August 18, 2016, http://circres.ahajournals.org/content/114/11/1804.full, doi:10.1161/CIRCRESAHA.114.302524. [This is second of a four-part thematic research series on The Autonomic Nervous System and the Cardiovascular System.—Ed.]

31. Thomas Cowan, "What Is the Real Cause of Heart Disease?" *Townsend Letter* 370 (May 20, 2014), accessed August 18, 2016, http://www.townsendletter.com. [With permission of *Townsend Letter*, this article was reprinted as "What's the Real Cause of Heart Attacks?" at http://articles.mercola.com/sites/articles/archive/2014/12/17/real-cause-heart-attacks.aspx.—Ed.]

32. Knut Sroka, "On the Genesis of Myocardial Ischemia," *Zeitschrift Fur Kardiologie* 93, no. 10 (October 2004): 768-83, accessed August 18, 2016, http://www.ncbi.nlm.nih.gov/pubmed/15492892, doi: 10.1007/s00392-004-0137-6.

33. Estela Kristal-Boneh et al., "Heart Rate Variability in Health and Disease," *Scandinavian Journal of Work, Environment and Health* 21, no. 2 (1995): 85-95, accessed August 18, 2016, http://www.ncbi.nlm.nih.gov/pubmed/7618063, doi:10.5271/sjweh.15.

34. Knut Sroka, C.J. Peimann, and H. Seevers, "Heart Rate Variability in Myocardial Ischemia During Daily Life," *Journal of Electrocardiology* 30, no. 1 (January 1997), May 11, 2005, accessed August 18, 2016, http://www.sciencedirect.com/science/article/pii/S0022073697800349, doi:10.1016/S0022-0736(97)80034-9.

35. James Scheuer and Norman Brachfeld, "Coronary Insufficiency: Relations Between Hemodynamic, Electrical, and Biochemical Parameters," *Circulation Research* 18 (February 1966): 178-89, accessed August 20, 2016, http://circres.ahajournals.org/content/18/2/178.full.pdf, doi:10.1161/01.RES.18.2.178.

36. Arnold M. Katz, "Effects of Ischemia on the Contractile Processes of Heart Muscle," *The American Journal of Cardiology* 32, no. 4 (September 20, 1973): 456-60, accessed August 21, 2016, www.ajconline.org/article/S0002-9149(73)80036-0/abstract, doi:10.1016/s0002-9149(73)80036-0.

37. Lorenzo Ghiadoni, et al., "Mental Stress Induces Transient Endothelial Dysfunction in Humans," *Circulation* 102, no. 20 (November 14, 2000): 2473-8, accessed August 21, 2016, http://circ.ahajournals.org/con-

tent/102/20/2473, doi:http://dx.doi.org/10.1161/01.CIR.102.20.2473

38. K.F. Harris and K.A. Matthews, "Interactions between Autonomic Nervous System Activity and Endothelial Function: A Model for the Development of Cardiovascular Disease," *Psychosomatic Medicine* 66, no. 2 (March/April 2004): 153-64, accessed August 21, 2016, http://www.ncbi.nlm.nih.gov/pubmed/15039499, doi: 10.1097/01.psy.0000116719.95524.e2.

39. P.C. Calder et al., "Inflammatory Disease Processes and Interactions with Nutrition," *British Journal of Nutrition* 101, no. S1 (May 2009): 1-45, accessed August 21, 2016, https://www.cambridge.org/core/journals/british-journal-of-nutrition/article/inflammatory-disease-processes-and-interactions-with-nutrition/8B6E145706102090539C4CE52A58F35E, doi:http://dx.doi.org/10.1017/S0007114509377867.

40. Alin Stirban, Thomas Gawlowski, and Michael Roden, "Vascular Effects of Advanced Glycation Endproducts: Clinical Effects and Molecular Mechanisms," *Molecular Metabolism* 3, no. 2 (April 2014): 94-108, December 7, 2013, accessed August 21, 2016, http://www.ncbi.nlm.nih.gov/pmc/articles/PMC3953708/pdf/main.pdf, doi:10.1016/j.molmet.2013.11.006.

41. F. William Danby, "Nutrition and Aging Skin: Sugar and Glycation," *Clinics in Dermatology* 28, no. 4 (July/August 2010): 409-11, accessed August 21, 2016, http://www.ncbi.nlm.nih.gov/pubmed/20620757, doi: 10.1016/j.clindermatol.2010.03.018.

42. Yori Gidron et al., "Vagus-Brain Communication in Atherosclerosis-Related Inflammation: A Neuroimmunomodulation Perspective of CAD," *Atherosclerosis* 195, no. 2 (December 2007): e1-e9, accessed August 22, 2016, http://www.sciencedirect.com/science/article/pii/S00 21915006006162?np=Y, doi: http://dx.doi.org/10.1016/j.atherosclerosis.2006.10.009.

43. Zara De Saint-Hilaire, et al., "Effects of a Bovine Alpha S1-Casein Tryptic Hydrolysate (CTH) on Sleep Disorder in Japanese General Population," *The Open Sleep Journal* 2 (May 15, 2009): 26-32, http://benthamopen.com/AB-STRACT/TOSLPJ-2-26, doi: 10.2174/1874620900902010026.

44. D. Lanoir et al., "Long Term Effects of a Bovine Milk Alpha-S1 Casein Hydrolysate on Healthy Low and High Stress Responders," in *Stress*, proceedings of World Congress on Stress, Edinburgh, Scotland, vol. 5: 124, (September 2002) accessed August 22, 2016, https://www.researchgate.net/publication/281783408_Long_term_effects_of_a_bovine_milk_alpha-S1-casein_hydrolysate_on_healthy_low_and_high_stress_responders.

45. M. Messaoudi, et al., "Effects of a Tryptic Hydrolysate from Bovine Milk αS1-casein on Hemodynamic Responses in Healthy Human Volunteers Facing Successive Mental and Physical Stress Situations," *European Journal of Nutrition* 44, no. 2 (March 2005): 128-32, November 2, 2004, accessed

ANM

August 22, 2016, http://www.ncbi.nlm.nih.gov/pubmed/15517308, doi: 10.1007/s00394-004-0534-7.

46. Izyaslav Lapin, "Phenibut (β-Phenyl-GABA): A Tranquilizer and Nootropic Drug," *CNS Drug Reviews* 7, no. 4 (December 2001): 471-81, accessed August 22, 2016, http://www.ncbi.nlm.nih.gov/pubmed/11830761.

47. Ratree Sudsuang, Vilai Chentanez, and Kongdej Veluvan, "Effect of Buddhist Meditation on Serum Cortisol and Total Protein Levels, Blood Pressure, Pulse Rate, Lung Volume and Reaction Time," *Physiology & Behavior* 50, no. 3 (September 1991): 543-48, accessed August 22, 2016, http://www.sciencedirect.com/science/article/pii/003193849190543W, doi:http://dx.doi.org/10.1016/0031-9384(91)90543-W.

48. Jon Kabat-Zinn, "An Outpatient Program in Behavioral Medicine for Chronic Pain Patients Based on the Practice of Mindfulness Meditation: Theoretical Considerations and Preliminary Results," *General Hospital Psychiatry* 4, no. 1 (April 1982): 33-47, accessed August 22, 2016, http://www.ncbi.nlm.nih.gov/pubmed/7042457, doi:10.1016/0163-8343(82)90026-3.

49. Sonia Sequeira, ed., "Special Issue: Advances in Meditation Research," in *Annals of the New York Academy of Sciences*, proceedings of 2015 Advances in Meditation Research conference, vol. 1373 (New York Academy of Sciences, June, 2016), 1-127, accessed August 22, 2016, http://www.nyas.org/publications/annals/Detail.aspx?cid=15fbb5d3-215c-40fe-a772-d8a71d00845e. [These 11 scholarly papers cover topics including mindfulness-based interventions for coping with cancer; the effects of mindfulness meditation on the immune system; mindfulness-based therapeutic approaches to remediate hedonic dysregulation in addiction, stress, and pain; promising links between meditation and brain preservation; the practice of yoga in school settings; mindfulness-based stress reduction and meditation as emerging tools to increase resilience; a nondual perspective on love and compassion meditation; transcending as a driver of development; an interoceptive map of central nervous system function and meditative mind–brain–body integration; mind wandering, mindful awareness, and mental tranquility; and a mechanistic account of mindfulness meditation–based pain relief.—Ed.)

50. R. P. Brown and P. L. Gerbarg, "Yoga Breathing, Meditation, and Longevity," *Annals of the New York Academy of Sciences* 1172 (August 2009): 54-62, accessed August 22, 2016, http://www.ncbi.nlm.nih.gov/pubmed/19735239, doi: 10.1111/j.1749-6632.2009.04394.x.

51. Nell Porter Brown, "Easing Ills through Tai Chi," *Harvard Magazine,* New England Regional, January/February 2010, accessed August 22, 2016, http://harvardmagazine.com/2010/01/researchers-study-tai-chi-benefits.

52. U.S. Centers for Disease Control and Prevention, "Alcohol and Public Health: Alcohol-related Disease Impact (ARDI)," (Alcohol Attributable

Deaths/United States/All Ages), accessed August 22, 2016, https://nccd.cdc.gov/DPH_ARDI/Default/Default.aspx.

53. U.S. Centers for Disease Control and Prevention (CDC), "Alcohol and Public Health: Fact Sheets - Underage Drinking," accessed August 22, 2016, http://www.cdc.gov/alcohol/fact-sheets/underage-drinking.htm.

54. U.S. Department of Transportation, National Highway Traffic Safety Administration, "Traffic Safety Facts: Young Drivers 2013 Data," accessed August 22, 2016, https://crashstats.nhtsa.dot.gov/Api/Public/ViewPublication/812200.

Chapter 3

No Citations

Chapter 4

1. Heinrich Wilhelm Dove, "Nachtrag zu den Combinationstonen" *Repertorium der Physik* 3 (Verlag Veit & Comp., Berlin, 1839): 404-405.

2. Gerald Oster, "Auditory Beats in the Brain," *Scientific American*, October 1, 1973, 94-102, accessed August 22, 2016, http://www.scientificamerican.com/article/auditory-beats-in-the-brain.

3. Robert A. Monroe, Method of and Apparatus for Inducing Desired States of Consciousness, U.S. Patent 5,356,368, issued October 18, 1994.

4. See note 2 above.

5. Shotaro Karino et al., "Neuromagnetic Responses to Binaural Beat in Human Cerebral Cortex," *Journal of Neurophysiology* 96, no. 4 (October 1, 2006): 1927-38, accessed August 25, 2016, http://jn.physiology.org/content/96/4/1927.long, doi: 10.1152/jn.00859.2005.

6. Rossitza Draganova et al., "Cortical Steady-state Responses to Central and Peripheral Auditory Beats," Cerebral Cortex 18, no. 5 (2008): 1193–1200, September 7, 2007, accessed August 25, 2016, http://cercor.oxfordjournals.org/content/18/5/1193.short, doi: 10.1093/cercor/bhm153.

7. Nantawachara Jirakittayakorn and Yodchanan Wongsawat, "The Brain Responses to Different Frequencies of Binaural Beat Sounds on QEEG at

Cortical Level," in proceedings of 2015 37th Annual International Conference of the Institute of Electrical and Electronics Engineers' Engineering in Medicine and Biology Society (EMBC), Milan, Italy, August 25-29, 2015, published online November 5, 2015, accessed August 25, 2016, http://ieeexplore.ieee.org/document/7319440, doi:10.1109/EMBC.2015.7319440.

8. Leila Chaieb et al., "Auditory Beat Stimulation and Its Effects on Cognition and Mood States," *Frontiers in Psychiatry* 6 (2015): 70, accessed August 25, 2016, http://www.ncbi.nlm.nih.gov/pmc/articles/PMC4428073, doi:10.3389/fpsyt.2015.00070.

9. Ibid.

10. "Stress & Brain Waves," The American Nutrition Association, October 31, 2009, accessed August 26, 2016, http://americannutritionassociation.org/node/257.

11. Fateme Dehghani-Arani, Reza Rostami, and Hosein Nadali, "Neurofeedback Training for Opiate Addiction: Improvement of Mental Health and Craving," *Applied Psychophysiology and Biofeedback* 38, no. 2 (June 2013): 133–141, April 20, 2013, accessed August 26, 2016, http://www.ncbi.nlm.nih.gov/pmc/articles/PMC3650238, doi:10.1007/s10484-013-9218-5.

12. Norman C. Moore, "A Review of EEG Biofeedback Treatment of Anxiety Disorders," *Clinical EEG and Neuroscience* 31, no. 1 (January 1, 2000): 1-6, accessed August 27, 2016, http://eeg.sagepub.com/content/31/1/1.extract, doi:10.1177/155005940003100105.

13. See note 8 above.

14. John H. Gruzelier, "A Theory of Alpha/theta Neurofeedback, Creative Performance Enhancement, Long Distance Functional Connectivity and Psychological Integration," *Cognitive Processing* 10, no. S1 (February 2009): 101-09, December 11, 2008, accessed August 27, 2016, http://www.ncbi.nlm.nih.gov/pubmed/19082646, doi: 10.1007/s10339-008-0248-5.

15. J. Stephen Bell, "The Use of EEG Theta Biofeedback in the Treatment of a Patient with Sleep-onset Insomnia," *Biofeedback and Self-Regulation* 4, no. 3 (September 1979): 229-36, http://www.ncbi.nlm.nih.gov/pubmed/486589, doi:10.1007/BF00998824.

16. Jean Aldini, *Essai Théorique Et Expérimental Sur Le Galvanisme* (Paris: Fournier Fils, 1804), accessed August 27, 2016, https://archive.org/stream/essaithoriqueete001aldi#page/n5/mode/2up.

17. Susan Southworth, "A Study of the Effects of Cranial Electrical Stimulation on Attention and Concentration," *Integrative Physiological and Behavioral Science* 34, no. 1 (January 1999): 43–53, accessed August 27, 2016, http://www.ncbi.nlm.nih.gov/pubmed/10381164, doi:10.1007/BF02688709.

18. Marc Auriacombe et al., "Transcutaneous Electrical Stimulation with Limoge Current Potentiates Morphine Analgesia and Attenuates Opiate Abstinence Syndrome," *Biological Psychiatry* 28, no. 8 (October 15, 1990): 650-656, accessed August 27, 2016, http://www.sciencedirect.com/science/article/pii/0006322390904517, doi:http://dx.doi.org/10.1016/0006-3223(90)90451-7.

19. Richard Schmitt et al., "Cranial Electrotherapy Stimulation Treatment of Cognitive Brain Dysfunction in Chemical Dependence," *Journal of Clinical Psychiatry* 45, no. 2 (February 1984): 60-63, accessed August 27, 2016, http://www.ncbi.nlm.nih.gov/pubmed/6363398.

20. Mauricio F. Villamar et al., "Noninvasive Brain Stimulation to Modulate Neuroplasticity in Traumatic Brain Injury," *Neuromodulation* 15, no. 4 (July/August 2012): 326-328, June 14, 2012, accessed August 28, 2016, http://www.ncbi.nlm.nih.gov/pubmed/22882244, doi:10.1111/j.1525-1403.2012.00474.x.

21. Ann Gill Taylor et al., "A Randomized, Controlled, Double-Blind Pilot Study of the Effects of Cranial Electrical Stimulation on Activity in Brain Pain Processing Regions in Individuals with Fibromyalgia," *Explore* 9, no. 1 (January/February 2013): 32-40, accessed August 28, 2016, http://www.sciencedirect.com/science/article/pii/S1550830712002169, doi:http://dx.doi.org/10.1016/j.explore.2012.10.006.

22. ADDitude Editors, "4 Brain Training Therapies for ADHD Children and Adults," *ADDitude Magazine*, Winter 2009, accessed August 28, 2016, http://www.additudemag.com/adhd/article/6563-2.html.

23. Alfred G. Bracciano et al., "Cranial Electrotheraphy Stimulation in the Treatment of Posttraumatic Stress Disorder: A Pilot Study of Two Military Veterans," *Journal of Neurotherapy* 16, no. 1 (2012): 60-69, March 2, 2012, accessed August 29, 2016, http://stress.org/wp-content/uploads/CES_Research/CES-for-PTSD.pdf, doi:10.1080/10874208.2012.650100.

24. Gad Alon et al., "Safety and Immediate Effect of Noninvasive Transcranial Pulsed Current Stimulation on Gait and Balance in Parkinson Disease," *Neurorehabilitation and Neural Repair* 26, no. 9 (May 2012): 1089-95, May 10, 2012, accessed August 29, 2016, http://www.ncbi.nlm.nih.gov/pubmed/22581566, doi: 10.1177/1545968312448233.

25. Min-Fang Kuo and Michael A. Nitsche, "Effects of Transcranial Electrical Stimulation on Cognition," *Clinical EEG and Neuroscience* 43, no. 3 (July 2012): 192-199, accessed August 29, 2016, http://eeg.sagepub.com/content/43/3/192.short, doi:10.1177/1550059412444975.

26. Mohammed Ferdjallah, Francis X. Bostick, Jr., and Ronald E. Barr "Potential and Current Density Distributions of Cranial Electrotherapy Stimulation (CES) in a Four-concentric-spheres Model," *IEEE Transactions on Biomedical Engineering* 43, no. 9 (September 1996): 939-43, accessed August 29, 2016,

http://www.ncbi.nlm.nih.gov/pubmed/9214809, doi:10.1109/10.532128.

27. R. L. Warner et al., "Transcranial Electrostimulation Effects on Rat Opioid and Neurotransmitter Levels," *Life Sciences* 54, no. 7 (1994): 481-490, accessed August 29, 2016, http://www.ncbi.nlm.nih.gov/pubmed/7906003, doi:10.1016/0024-3205(94)00407-2.

28. G. Blake Holloway, Systems and Methods for Balancing and Maintaining the Health of the Human Autonomic Nervous System, U.S. Patent 9,079,030, filed June 16, 2011, and issued July 14, 2015.

29. National Institutes of Health, National Institute of Mental Health, *Brain Basics: The Working Brain*, accessed August 29, 2016, http://www.nimh.nih.gov/health/educational-resources/brain-basics/brain-basics.shtml.

30. Marty Hinz, Alvin Stein, and Thomas Uncini, "Relative Nutritional Deficiencies Associated with Centrally Acting Monomines," *International Journal of General Medicine* 5 (May 8, 2012): 413-30, accessed August 29, 2016, http://www.ncbi.nlm.nih.gov/pmc/articles/PMC3355850, doi:10.2147/IJGM.S31179.

31. J. M. Everett et al., "Theanine Consumption, Stress and Anxiety in Human Clinical Trials: A Systematic Review," *Journal of Nutrition and Intermediary Metabolism* 4 (June 2016): 41-42, accessed August 29, 2016, http://www.sciencedirect.com/science/article/pii/S2352385915003138, doi:http://dx.doi.org/10.1016/j.jnim.2015.12.308.

32. C. V. Russoniello et al., "Heart Rate Variability and Biological Age: Implications for Health and Gaming," *Cyberpsychology, Behavior and Social Networking* 4 (April 16, 2013), accessed August 29, 2016, http://www.ncbi.nlm.nih.gov/pubmed/23574369, doi:10.1089/cyber.2013.1505.

33. Rachel Lampert et al., "Decreased Heart Rate Variability Is Associated With Higher Levels of Inflammation in Middle-Aged Men," *American Heart Journal* 156, no. 4 (October 2008): 759.e1-759e.7, accessed August 29, 2016, http://www.ncbi.nlm.nih.gov/pubmed/18926158, doi:10.1016/j.ahj.2008.07.009.

34. Robert G. Robinson et al., "Decreased Heart Rate Variability Is Associated with Poststroke Depression," *The American Journal of Geriatric Psychiatry: Official Journal of the American Association for Geriatric Psychiatry* 16, no. 11 (November 2008): 867–873, accessed August 29, 2016, http://www.ncbi.nlm.nih.gov/pmc/articles/PMC2621363, doi:10.1097/JGP.0b013e318180057d.

35. John A. Chalmers et al., "Anxiety Disorders Are Associated with Reduced Heart Rate Variability: A Meta-Analysis," *Frontiers in Psychiatry* 5 (July 11, 2014): 80, accessed August 29, 2016, http://www.ncbi.nlm.nih.gov/pubmed/25071612, doi:10.3389/fpsyt.2014.00080.

36. P. K. Stein and R. E. Kleiger, "Insights from the Study of Heart Rate Variability," *Annual Review of Medicine* 50 (1999): 249-61, accessed August 29, 2016, http://www.ncbi.nlm.nih.gov/pubmed/10073276, doi:10.1146/annurev.med.50.1.249.

37. Task Force of the European Society of Cardiology and the North American Society of Pacing and Electrophysiology, "Heart Rate Variability: Standards of Measurement, Physiological Interpretation and Clinical Use," *Circulation* 93, no. 5 (March 1, 1996): 1043-65, accessed August 29, 2016, http://www.ncbi.nlm.nih.gov/pubmed/8598068, doi:http://dx.doi.org/10.1161/01 CIR.93.5.1043.

Chapter 5

1. Sheldon Cohen, Denise Janicki-Deverts, and Gregory E. Miller, "Psychological Stress and Disease," *Journal of the American Medical Association* 298, no. 14 (October 10, 2007): 1685-87, accessed August 30, 2016, http://www.psy.cmu.edu/~scohen/JAMA_2007_Psy_Stress_Disease.pdf, doi: 10.1001/jama.298.14.1685.

2. Mayo Clinic Staff, "Chronic Stress Puts Your Health at Risk," Mayo Clinic, April 21, 2016, accessed August 30, 2016, http://www.mayoclinic.org/healthy-lifestyle/stress-management/in-depth/stress/art-20046037?pg=1 Anxiety.

3. Elizabeth Agnvall, "Stress! Don't Let It Make You Sick," *AARP Bulletin*, November 2014, accessed August 30, 2016, http://www.aarp.org/health/healthy-living/info-2014/stress-and-disease.html.

4. See note 1 above.

5. Mary Franz, "Nutrition, Inflammation, and Disease," *Today's Dietitian*, February 2014, 44, accessed August 30, 2016, http://www.todaysdietitian.com/newarchives/020314p44.shtml.

6. Ibid.

7. F. Sardi et al., "Alzheimer's Disease, Autoimmunity and Inflammation. The Good, the Bad and the Ugly," *Autoimmunity Reviews* 11, no. 2 (December 2011): 149-53, October 5, 2011, accessed August 30, 2016, http://www.ncbi.nlm.nih.gov/pubmed/21996556, doi: 10.1016/j.autrev.2011.09.005.

8. Sharon Palmer, "Is There a Link Between Nutrition and Autoimmune Disease?," *Today's Dietitian*, November 2011, 36, accessed August 30, 2016, http://www.todaysdietitian.com/newarchives/110211p36.shtml.

9. See note 5 above.

10. H. Lu, W. Ouyang, and C. Huang, "Inflammation, a Key Event in Cancer Development," *Molecular Cancer Research* 4, no. 4 (April 2006): accessed August 30, 2016, http://www.ncbi.nlm.nih.gov/pubmed/16603636, doi:10.1158/1541-7786.MCR-05-0261.

11. Sandor Szabo, Yvette Tache, and Arpad Somogyi, "The Legacy of Hans Selye and the Origins of Stress Research: A Retrospective 75 Years after His Landmark Brief "letter" to the Editor of Nature," *Stress: The International Journal on the Biology of Stress* 15, no. 5 (September 2012), accessed August 30, 2016, http://www.tandfonline.com/doi/abs/10.3109/10253890.2012.710919?journalCode=ists20, doi:http://dx.doi.org/10.3109/10253890.2012.710919.

12. Gregory E. Miller, Edith Chen, and Eric S. Zhou, "If It Goes Up, Must It Come Down? Chronic Stress and the Hypothalamic-pituitary-adrenocortical Axis in Humans," *Psychological Bulletin* 133, no. 1 (January 2007): 25-45, accessed August 30, 2016, http://www.ncbi.nlm.nih.gov/pubmed/17201569, doi:http://dx.doi.org/10.1037/0033-2909.133.1.25.

13. National Institutes of Health, National Cancer Institute, "Leading Causes of Death in US, 1975 vs 2013 Percent of All Causes of Death," *SEER Cancer Statistics Review: 1975-2013*, accessed August 30, 2016, http://seer.cancer.gov/csr/1975_2013/results_merged/topic_lead_cod.pdf.

14. "Lifetime Risk of Developing or Dying From Cancer," American Cancer Society, March 23, 2016, accessed August 30, 2016, http://www.cancer.org/cancer/cancerbasics/lifetime-probability-of-developing-or-dying-from-cancer.

15. Hyunsoon Cho et al., "When Do Changes in Cancer Survival Mean Progress? The Insight From Population Incidence and Mortality," *Journal of the National Cancer Institute. Monographs.* 2014, no. 49 (November 2014): 87–197, accessed August 30, 2016, http://jncimono.oxfordjournals.org/content/2014/49/187.long, doi:10.1093/jncimonographs/lgu014.

16. National Institutes of Health, National Cancer Institute, "NCI Budget and Appropriations," April 19, 2016, accessed August 30, 2016, https://www.cancer.gov/about-nci/budget.

17. American Cancer Society, "Current Grants by Cancer Type," August 1, 2016, accessed August 30, 2016, http://www.cancer.org/research/currentlyfundedcancerresearch/grants-by-cancer-type.

18. See note 10 above.

19. Helen Lavretsky, Martha Sajatovic, and Charles Reynolds, III, eds., *Complementary and Integrative Therapies for Mental Health and Aging*, 1st ed. (New York: Oxford University Press, 2016).

20. American Heart Association, "Heart Disease and Stroke — At-A-Glance," December 2014, accessed August 30, 2016, https://www.heart.org/idc/groups/ahamah-public/@wcm/@sop/@smd/documents/downloadable/ucm_470704.pdf.

21. Centers for Disease Control and Prevention, "Women and Heart Disease Fact Sheet," June 16, 2016, accessed August 30, 2016, http://www.cdc.gov/dhdsp/data_statistics/fact_sheets/fs_women_heart.htm.

22. Centers for Disease Control and Prevention, "High Blood Pressure Fact Sheet," June 16, 2016, accessed August 30, 2016, http://www.cdc.gov/dhdsp/data_statistics/fact_sheets/fs_bloodpressure.htm.

23. James J. DiNicolantonio, Sean C. Lucan, and James H. O'Keefe, "The Evidence for Saturated Fat and For Sugar Related to Coronary Heart Disease," *Progress in Cardiovascular Diseases* 58, no. 5 (March/April 2016): 464-72, November 14, 2015, accessed August 30, 2016, http://www.ncbi.nlm.nih.gov/pubmed/26586275, doi:10.1016/j.pcad.2015.11.006.

24. Barbara H. Roberts, *The Truth about Statins: Risks and Alternatives to Cholesterol-lowering Drugs* (New York: Gallery Books, 2012), accessed August 30, 2016, http://www.simonandschuster.com/books/The-Truth-About-Statins/Barbara-H-Roberts/9781451656398.

25. Mark R. Goldstein and Luca Mascitelli, "Do Statins Cause Diabetes?," *Current Diabetes Reports* 13, no. 3 (June 2013): 381-90, accessed August 30, 2016, http://www.ncbi.nlm.nih.gov/pubmed/23456437#, doi:10.1007/s11892-013-0368-x.

26. Tim Assimes, "International Study Points to Inflammation as Cause of Plaque Buildup in Heart Vessels, Researchers Say," Stanford University News Center, December 2, 2012, accessed August 31, 2016, http://med.stanford.edu/news/all-news/2012/12/international-study-points-to-inflammation-as-cause-of-plaque-buildup-in-heart-vessels-researchers-say.html.

27. Paul M. Ridker et al., "Comparison of C-Reactive Protein and Low-Density Lipoprotein Cholesterol Levels in the Prediction of First Cardiovascular Events," *The New England Journal of Medicine* 347 (November 14, 2002): 1557-1565, accessed August 31, 2016, http://www.nejm.org/doi/full/10.1056/NEJMoa021993, doi:10.1056/NEJMoa021993.

28. Harvard Medical School, "What You Eat Can Fuel or Cool Inflammation, a Key Driver of Heart Disease, Diabetes, and Other Chronic Conditions," *Harvard Health Publications*, February 2007, accessed August 31, 2016, http://www.health.harvard.edu/family-health-guide/what-you-eat-can-fuel-or-cool-inflammation-a-key-driver-of-heart-disease-diabetes-and-other-chronic-conditions.

29. Lena Jonasson et al., "Advice to Follow a Low-carbohydrate Diet Has a Favourable Impact on Low-grade Inflammation in Type 2 Diabetes Compared with Advice to Follow a Low-fat Diet," *Annals of Medicine* 46, no. 3 (2014): 182-87, April 30, 2014, accessed August 31, 2016, http://www.tandfonline.com/doi/full/10.3109/07853890.2014.894286, http://dx.doi.org/10.3 109/07853890.2014.894286.

30. Tian Hu et al., "The Effects of a Low-Carbohydrate Diet vs. a Low-Fat Diet on Novel Cardiovascular Risk Factors: A Randomized Controlled Trial," *Nutrients* 7, no. 9 (September 17, 2015): 7978-94, accessed August 31, 2016, http://www.ncbi.nlm.nih.gov/pubmed/26393645, doi:10.3390/nu7095377.

31. See Cowen, Chapter 2 note 31.

32. Brian Olshansky et al., "Parasympathetic Nervous System and Heart Failure: Pathophysiology and Potential Implications for Therapy," *Circulation* 118, no. 8 (August 19, 2008): 863-71, accessed August 31, 2016, http://circ.ahajournals.org/content/118/8/863.long, doi:http://dx.doi.org/10.1161/CIRCULATIONAHA.107.760405.

33. Takuya Kishi, "Heart Failure as an Autonomic Nervous System Dysfunction," *Journal of Cardiology* 59, no. 2 (March 2012): 117-22, accessed August 31, 2016, http://www.ncbi.nlm.nih.gov/pubmed/22341431, doi:10.1016/j.jjcc.2011.12.006.

34. See Cowan, Chapter 2 note 31.

35. Thomas M. Heffron, "Insomnia Awareness Day Facts and Stats," American Academy of Sleep Medicine, March 10, 2014, accessed August 31, 2016, http://www.sleepeducation.org/news/2014/03/10/insomnia-awareness-day-facts-and-stats.

36. Division of Sleep Medicine, Harvard Medical School, "Sleep and Disease Risk," Healthy Sleep, December 18, 2008, accessed August 31, 2016, http://healthysleep.med.harvard.edu/healthy/matters/consequences/sleep-and-disease-risk.

37. Ann Pietrangelo, "The Effects of Sleep Deprivation on the Body," Healthline, August 19, 2014, accessed August 31, 2016, http://www.healthline.com/health/sleep-deprivation/effects-on-body.

38. See Holloway, Chapter 4 note 28.

39. J.K. Kiecolt-Glaser et al., "Slowing of Wound Healing by Psychological Stress," *Lancet* 346, no. 8984 (November 4, 1995): 1194-6, accessed August 31, 2016, http://www.ncbi.nlm.nih.gov/pubmed/7475659.

Chapter 6

No Citations

About the Authors

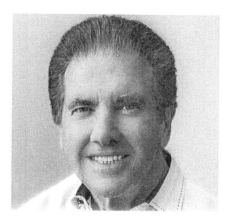

Michael Galitzer, M.D.

Dr. Michael Galitzer is a nationally recognized expert in energy medicine, integrative medicine and bio-identical hormone replacement therapy, as well as a co-author of *Outstanding Health: The 6 Essential Keys to Maximize Your Energy and Well Being*. For more than 40 years, Dr. Galitzer has been a leading figure and innovator in the field of longevity, or anti-aging medicine.

Dr. Galitzer graduated from the State University of New York Upstate Medical Center, and moved in 1973 to Los Angeles, where he practiced emergency medicine for 15 years. He was among the first 100 doctors in the U.S. to become board certified in emergency medicine. Eventually, Dr. Galitzer began studying integrative medicine, including herbs, nutrition, energy medicine and homeopathy. In 1990, he completed a course in medical acupuncture and incorporated it into his private practice established in 1987 at Santa Monica, California.

Dr. Galitzer utilizes revolutionary treatments to produce remarkable and rapid improvements in his patients' health and vitality. He draws from both traditional and complementary medicine, including sound and light therapy, toxin elimination and intravenous supplementation. His patient list includes many top figures from Hollywood, business and sports, as well as people from across North and South America, Europe, Asia, Africa and Australia.

Dr. Galitzer has been a member of the American Association of Medical Acupuncture, the American Association of Acupuncture and Bio-Energetic Medicine, the International Oxidative Medical Association and the American Academy of Anti-Aging Medicine. He was a board member of the American College for Advancement in

Medicine, a leading organization of physicians in the field of alternative and complementary medicine. He has given lectures all over the world on longevity, as well as alternative and bio-energetic medicine.

For the past decade, Dr. Galitzer has been a featured contributor to nine bestselling books by actress, author and health advocate Suzanne Somers. They include:

• *I'm Too Young for This!: The Natural Hormone Solution to Enjoy Perimenopause (2014)*

• *Bombshell: Explosive Medical Secrets that Will Redefine Aging 2012)*

• *Sexy Forever: How to Fight Fat After Forty (2010)*

• *Knockout: Interviews with Doctors Who are Curing Cancer— and How to Prevent Getting It in the First Place (2009)*

• Breakthrough: Eight Steps to Wellness (2008)

• *Ageless: The Naked Truth About Bioidentical Hormones (2007)*

• *The Sexy Years: Discover the Hormone Connection: The Secret to Fabulous Sex, Great Health, and Vitality, for Women and Men (2004).*

In addition to *Outstanding Health,* Dr. Galitzer's other publications include "Re-ignite Your Spark, No Batteries Required," a chapter on bioidentical hormones in *Alternative Medicine, the Definitive Guide (2002),* and research papers published in *Explore Magazine* and *The Townsend Letter for Doctors.* His work has been featured in articles in the *New York Times Magazine, USA Today* and *C Magazine* of California.

In addition to his thriving practice in Santa Monica, Dr. Galitzer is the medical director of The American Health Institute in Los Angeles, an organization dedicated to education and research in the areas of energy medicine and cancer. He currently resides in Los Angeles, with his wife and four children.

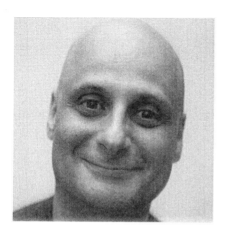

Larry Trivieri Jr.

Larry Trivieri Jr. is a bestselling author and a nationally recognized lay authority on holistic, integrative and non-drug-based healing methods. For more than 30 years, he has explored techniques for optimal wellness and human transformation, including acid-alkaline balance. Trivieri has interviewed and studied with more than 400 of the world's top physicians and health practitioners in over 50 disciplines of holistic health.

Trivieri is the author or co-author of more than 20 books on health, including *The Acid-Alkaline Lifestyle, The Acid-Alkaline Food Guide, Juice Alive, The American Holistic Medical Association Guide to Holistic Health, The Self-Care Guide to Holistic Medicine,* and *Health On The Edge: Visionary Views of Healing in the New Millennium.* With Dr. Michael Galitzer, he co-authored *Outstanding Health: The 6 Essential Keys To Maximize Your Energy and Well Being.*

He was editor and principal writer of both editions of the landmark health encyclopedia, *Alternative Medicine: The Definitive Guide,* and has written over 200 articles for internet-based health sites, including 1HealthyWorld.com and IntegrativeHealthReview.com. He has written numerous feature articles for publications, including *Alternative Medicine* (for which he also served as contributing editor from 1999 to 2002), *Natural Health, Natural Solutions* and *Yoga Journal.* Articles about him have appeared in a number of national publications, including *The Washington Post.* As an author of children's novels, Trivieri has penned *The Monster and Freddie Fype* and *Krystle's Quest.*

Trivieri is dedicated to helping usher in a new era of wellness and health care in the 21st century by sharing his accumulated wealth of potentially life-saving information with as wide an audience as possible. To that end, he lectures about health and has been a featured guest on numerous television and radio shows across the United States. He resides in upstate New York.